WORKBOOK TO ACCO~~I~~

FOUNDATIONS OF RESPIRATORY CARE

Second Edition

Written by
William French and Lisa Schmuck

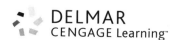

DELMAR
CENGAGE Learning™

Australia • Brazil • Japan • Korea • Mexico • Singapore • Spain • United Kingdom • United States

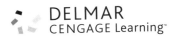
DELMAR
CENGAGE Learning™

Workbook to Accompany Foundations of Respiratory Care, Second Edition
William French and Lisa Schmuck

Vice President, Editorial: Dave Garza

Director of Learning Solutions: Matthew Kane

Associate Acquisitions Editor: Christina Gifford

Managing Editor: Marah Bellegarde

Senior Product Manager: Darcy M. Scelsi

Editorial Assistant: Nicole Manikas

Vice President, Marketing: Jennifer Ann Baker

Associate Marketing Manager: Johnathan Sheehan

Senior Production Director: Wendy A. Troeger

Production Manager: Andrew Crouth

Content Project Manager: Brooke Greenhouse

Senior Art Director: David Arsenault

Library of Congress Control Number: 2011934924

ISBN-13: 978-1-4354-6987-7

ISBN-10: 1-4354-6987-9

Delmar
5 Maxwell Drive
Clifton Park, NY 12065-2919
USA

Cengage Learning is a leading provider of customized learning solutions with office locations around the globe, including Singapore, the United Kingdom, Australia, Mexico, Brazil, and Japan. Locate your local office at:
international.cengage.com/region

Cengage Learning products are represented in Canada by Nelson Education, Ltd.

To learn more about Delmar, visit **www.cengage.com/delmar**

Purchase any of our products at your local college store or at our preferred online store **www.cengagebrain.com**

Notice to the Reader
Publisher does not warrant or guarantee any of the products described herein or perform any independent analysis in connection with any of the product information contained herein. Publisher does not assume, and expressly disclaims, any obligation to obtain and include information other than that provided to it by the manufacturer. The reader is expressly warned to consider and adopt all safety precautions that might be indicated by the activities described herein and to avoid all potential hazards. By following the instructions contained herein, the reader willingly assumes all risks in connection with such instructions. The publisher makes no representations or warranties of any kind, including but not limited to, the warranties of fitness for particular purpose or merchantability, nor are any such representations implied with respect to the material set forth herein, and the publisher takes no responsibility with respect to such material. The publisher shall not be liable for any special, consequential, or exemplary damages resulting, in whole or part, from the readers' use of, or reliance upon, this material.

Printed in the United States of America
1 2 3 4 5 6 7 15 14 13 12 11

CONTENTS

Scope of Practice

The History and Scope of Respiratory Care

INTRODUCTION

Respiratory care practice is an emerging profession, but its roots extend back thousands of years to the works of Hippocrates, Aristotle, and Galen. Not until the 1600s did the role of oxygen begin to be understood. William Harvey demonstrated blood circulation. Robert Boyle elucidated the volume and pressure relationships of gases. Joseph Priestley experimentally produced oxygen. In the 1700s, Antoine Lavoisier gave oxygen its name and correctly described the basic physiology of respiration. Thomas Beddoes established the Pneumatic Institute of Bristol, England, and was the first to use oxygen therapeutically. Growth of the field of respiratory care burgeoned in the twentieth century with rapid advancements in science and technology, many of which resulted from research in World Wars I and II.

Over the years, the role of persons who delivered oxygen therapy changed from mere equipment technicians (oxygen orderlies) to fully accredited allied health-care providers. A national professional organization developed a set of standards for requirements, education, and scope of practice.

Implementation of evidence-based practices and the refinement of protocol-based care methods will, without a doubt, continue to expand the scope of practice. They will lead to the advancement of the respiratory care practitioner's ability to provide timely and efficacious patient care with reduced morbidity and mortality. They will also enhance the potential for developing effective multidisciplinary care teams.

Future health-care reform in the United States will pose many challenges to the field of respiratory care as the government attempts to contain rising prices while preserving and increasing access for citizens. The leadership of the specialty will need to be especially nimble in negotiating each of the legislative changes that affect practice sites.

Discussion Activities and Questions

1. Define profession in your own terms. What are some characteristics of a profession?

Profession, by definition covers a wide spectrum of areas. In general, a profession is any type of work that one attributes to themself. However, it usually is used to describe a higher level of job placement. An example would be a lawyer or a physician.

2. What are some professions within the health-care system? *Professions in the health-care system would be physicians, nurses, anesthesiologists, physical therapists, respiratory therapists for example.*

3. Discuss what attracted you to the respiratory care profession (as opposed to other health-care professions). *My grandfather suffered with cardio pulmonary issues for years. He was a smoker and I saw how he struggled in his last few years of life. I would like to go to work every day and educate people to improve their quality of life and to make a difference in patient care.*

4. Create a timeline for the significant discoveries related to pulmonary medicine.

5. Create a timeline for respiratory care from its origin to the present.

6. Discuss what is meant by "scope of practice." *There have been laws put into place over time to define the practice of Respiratory Therapy. The "scope of practice" really provides a description of duties that an RRT could practice and the minimum amount of credentialling that would be accepted.*

7. Discuss and list different forms of advanced credentials for respiratory therapists (e.g., ACLS, PALS, NRP, etc.).

Thought Questions

1. Should medicine be directed toward ending disease? *Medicine should be directed at ending disease. I feel that treatment is not quite enough. If health care is practicing to make a patient feel better for the time being, but not giving therapy along with education, the future of health care would not be so bright. Getting people well should be the ultimate goal.*

2. What is the difference between Medicare and Medicaid? *Medicare provides assistance to pay for health services for people 65 and older and for persons who have been recieving social security disability benefits for 2 yrs. medicaid authorizes federal matching funds to assist the states in providing health care for certain income groups at or near the federal poverty line.*

3. What do you believe is the impact of switching from fee-for-service to PPS? *PPS focus was mostly about hospital costs, so because patients in the hospital were recieving less care and shorter hospital stays, there was a boom in clinic and outside facility care. Respiratory Therapists also became needed outside of hospitals, so the scope of practice increased.*

4. How do you believe managed care has affected and will affect respiratory care? *The cost of care is on the rise as it has been for a long time. The greatest dilemma in respiratory will be to continue to give the necessary care to patients in conjunction with a system trying to contain cost. The patients will be affected by either the services provided and care they recieve or not be able to afford health care.*

REVIEW

True or False

T 1. Respiratory therapists are often included on rapid response teams.

T 2. The Joint Commission includes respiratory therapists on the Professional Technical Advisory Committee.

F 3. "Acuity level" refers to length of stay in an acute care hospital.

Multiple Choice

1. In 1944, who authored the first textbook in what was then called inhalation therapy?

   a. Dr. Donald Egan
   b. Dr. John Severinghaus
   c. Mr. Jimmy Young
   (d.) Dr. Alvin Barach

2. Which of the following is credited with the first therapeutic use of oxygen?

   a. Joseph Priestley
   (b.) Thomas Beddoes
   c. William Harvey
   d. Alvin Barach

3. Which of the following is considered the father of Western medicine?

   (a.) Hippocrates
   b. Galen
   c. Socrates
   d. Vesalius

4. Which of the following is a fiduciary?

   a. legal official
   b. patient
   c. director
   (d.) trustee

5. In what year was the Inhalation Therapy Association formed?

   (a.) 1947
   b. 1952
   c. 1959
   d. 1965

6. Which of the following agencies currently accredits schools of respiratory care?

   a. NBRC
   b. Joint Commission
   (c.) CoARC
   d. AARC

7. Since the 1990s, the advent of which of the following has greatly affected all facets of health care?

   a. Medicare
   (b.) managed care
   c. prospective payment
   d. insurance reform

Legal, Professional, and Ethical Practice

INTRODUCTION

Respiratory care is a clinical practice and for the most part our careers are involved with technical and scientific issues. However, in order to truly be successful in practice, RTs must ensure that our performance is not only technically correct but also legally, ethically, and professionally correct. As health-care providers, RTs draw from a vast well of trust that has been formed by the past practices of the specialists who have come before us. The patient's trust—that the provider is working single-mindedly on his or her behalf, that there are no conflicts of interest, that no secrets are being hidden, and that the provider's behavior is both ethical and legal—is an important part of the therapeutic relationship.

The provision of ethical and legal practice is not negotiable; it cannot be set aside because of schedules or personal preference or in an effort to be more efficient or productive. Performing ethically and legally is not just a nice way to practice; it is the only way to practice. In some sense, ethical, lawful behavior lies at the very heart of what is meant by being professional.

Discussion Activities and Questions

1. What is the difference between legal requirements and professional etiquette? *The laws are the main difference between legal requirements and professional etiquette. The laws govern what is acceptable and what is not. Professional etiquette is how you carry yourself in attitude and appearance as a professional.*

2. List four common legal issues in everyday life.
   1. use of drugs and/or alcohol
   2. conflicts of interest
   3. Falsification of credentials
   4. Performing non-prescribed services

3. List four common ethical issues.

Confidentiality
Veracity
autonomy
beneficence

4. Give some examples of torts that may apply to the provision of health care. If a doctor ordered a therapist to give a treatment or a medicine and they were neglegent in doing so and this caused harm to a patient. Another example would be using force with a patient or having them do something that they did not consent to.

5. Give some examples of slander. If a nurse or therapist was talking about a physician in a negative way and through hear say, that physician's reputation with their patients may suffer. another example would be stating that a certain person does not do a good job because some one told you something That was not true.

6. What are the four classes of tort actions involving invasion of privacy?

1. Presenting someone in a false light to the public
2. misappropriation
3. Intrusion
4. Public disclosure

7. Discuss and give some examples of double effect as it applies to respiratory care. Double effect is when someone is faced with a situation that is positive in one way yet negative in another.

8. Discuss how an individual's religious beliefs might affect his or her medical treatment. There are many religions that do not allow certain practices in medicine. as a health-care worker, we should expect that there may be times that a person refuses a medicine or treatment based upon their personal religious beliefs. Even if the medicine or treatment is necessary, it is the patients right to decide.

9. Define "law."

a law is something that is set as a rule for which someone would obligate themself to abide by in some way.

10. What is the AARC Statement of Ethics and Professional Conduct? How will it apply to you as a clinician?

The AARC statement of Ethics & Professional Conduct are a set of ethical guidelines to which an RRT must abide. It is a list of important principles that must remain a constant set of reminders. I have always and plan to follow these guidelines and as a rule, ask myself how I would wish to be treated.

Thought Questions

1. In your respiratory therapy program, what is the primary basis for how your clinical/professional competency is assessed?

2. Jim is the respiratory therapist assigned to the ED. He receives a call to draw arterial blood on a 25-year-old female admitted for shortness of breath of recent onset. Upon arrival, Jim introduces himself and explains what he is there to do. The patient refuses the procedure.

   a. What should Jim do at this point?

   b. What would be the problem if Jim restrained the patient and attempted the procedure even though she had refused it?

3. Jane is the RT assigned to the ED. She receives a stat call. Upon arrival, she is asked to participate in the intubation of a suspected drug overdose. After a moment, she recognizes the patient as being a well-known celebrity. Does she have the right to tell anyone outside of the ED? Why or why not? What if the patient was a distant relative?

4. David is summoned to the ED to help with a patient who was transported by the local paramedics because of a self-inflicted gunshot wound. Does David have the right to refuse to help care for this patient? Why or why not? What if the patient was shot by the police after he killed another person?

5. A wealthy business owner needs cardiac surgery. The hospital is currently very busy and the business owner is medically stable at the moment. Is it acceptable for him to be placed ahead of other patients with similar medical situations if he offers to pay extra for the procedure or donate a significant sum to the hospital? Why or why not?

6. The respiratory therapist is working with a 52-year-old patient who experienced a massive CVA and is currently in ICU on mechanical ventilation. The RT has heard that the probable prognosis is sustained coma and that the patient will need to be transferred to a long-term care facility. However, the attending physician has not yet informed the family. What should the RT do or say if the patient's family asks about the patient's status?

REVIEW

True or False

F 1. Incomplete patient records is an example of a common ethical issue.

I 2. Performing nonprescribed services is an example of a common legal issue.

I 3. A misdemeanor is a crime usually punished by incarceration for less than one year.

I 4. Private law deals with definition, regulation, and enforcement of rights in cases between citizen and citizen.

I 5. Respondeat superior means "let the master speak."

F 6. During a jury trial, the defendant has a burden of proof.

F 7. The patient must always give informed consent before undergoing any medical treatment or intervention.

I 8. A patient may refuse any recommended treatment.

Multiple Choice

1. Which of the following is a possible sanction for an ethics violation?

   a. loss of professional credentials
   b. loss of professional reputation
   c. loss of license
   d. termination of employment

2. Which of the following is the most fundamental principle of law?

   a. concern for justice and fairness
   b. plasticity and change
   c. doctrine of personal responsibility
   d. administration of sanctions

3. Which of the following are elements of U.S. law derived from those of Great Britain?

   1. trial by jury
   2. professional judiciary
   3. incarceration for offenses
   4. interpretation of case law

   a. 1, 2
   b. 1, 2, 4
   c. 2, 3
   d. 3, 4

4. Which of the following is the primary source of common law?

   a. legislative action
   b. administrative decree
   c. case law
   d. trial by jury

5. Which of the following best describes statutory law?

   a. decisions created by judicial activism
   b. statutes created by the legislative branch
   c. rules enacted by decree
   d. rules adapted from previous laws

6. Practice acts are examples of which of the following?

   a. common law
   b. administrative mandate
   c. judicial decision
   d. statutory law

7. Typically, practice acts address which of the following elements?

  1. professional nomenclature
  2. scope of practice
  3. exemption
  4. grounds for administrative action

  a. 1, 3
  b. 1, 2, 4

  c. 2, 4
  d. 2, 3, 4

8. A respiratory therapist is participating in resuscitation of a patient who was brought into the ED because of methamphetamine overdose. During the resuscitation, the RT frequently refers to the patient with terms such as "tweaker" and other blatantly derogatory epithets. This is an example of which of the following?

  a. slander
  b. assault

  c. libel
  d. violation of professional etiquette

9. In X Hospital, all patients receive the same treatment regardless of their means, ability to pay, or social standing. This is an example of which of the following?

  a. procedural justice
  b. socialism

  c. fragmented health care
  d. distributive justice

10. Using virtue ethics, the respiratory therapist is guided by which of the following?

  a. duty-oriented decision making
  b. tradition of earlier practitioners

  c. policies and procedures
  d. divine command

The Applied Sciences

CHAPTER 3

Applied Physics

INTRODUCTION

Physics, especially of fluids and gas, is among the most useful studies a respiratory therapist can undertake. An in-depth understanding of the principles of physics enables the respiratory therapist to understand the interactions among physics, physiology, and pathophysiology. In addition to the gas laws, the laws governing electricity, elasticity, force, and motion are all relevant to respiratory care. The respiratory therapist must be competent in the use of scientific notation, the metric system, and dimensional analysis, because the solving of physiological equations plays a large part in the science of respiratory care.

As experts in the application of technology to the seriously ill or recovering patient, respiratory specialists must understand how both patient and equipment work and interact if they are to be at the peak of their profession. Having a grasp of physical principles and their application to both technology and humanity is a never-ending duty owed to patients. Many people understand physics and many understand patients, but relatively few understand how to manage the interface where patient and technology meet. That is the respiratory therapist's skill.

Discussion Activities and Questions

1. What is the difference between a theory and a principle?

2. What is the purpose of dimensional analysis?

3. Define inertia according to Newton's first law. Think of some examples of a body at rest and a body in uniform motion.

4. What happens to the compliance of a balloon as you inflate it, starting when it is completely collapsed and continuing to maximum expansion? How does this apply to the lung? (This is an easy experiment to try.)

5. Explain the difference between mass and weight. Can you think of any instances in which the difference might be important?

6. List at least four devices used in respiratory therapy that operate on electricity.

7. People with obstructive sleep apnea often use a continuous positive airway pressure (CPAP) machine. A patient who is in the hospital for hip surgery wants to bring in his CPAP machine from home. What should the hospital do about this? (This is a point of controversy in many hospitals.)

8. How would the viscosity of mucus affect the ability of the lung to remove it? How would this affect what you do as a respiratory therapist?

9. Using Poiseuille's law, would replacing an endotracheal tube with a tracheostomy tube decrease resistance to gas flow into the lower airway? Why or why not?

10. In the tracheobronchial tree, the flow of gas is most laminar in the terminal bronchioles. Why?

11. Explain how the Bernoulli principle differs from the Venturi principle.

12. Explain how Boyle's law applies to normal ventilation.

13. It is often said that you should not measure the pressure in your tires right after you have driven the car a long distance. Why not?

14. Using Dalton's law, what happens to the partial pressure of oxygen (PO_2) as you move to higher elevations?

15. Babies born before 32 weeks gestation often lack surfactant, which causes their work of breathing to increase. Using LaPlace's law, explain why.

REVIEW

True or False

___T___ 1. Occam's Razor states: When given a choice of solutions, select the obvious one.

___F___ 2. Newton's second law states: For every action, there is an equal but opposite reaction.

___F___ 3. Electricity is the flow of electrons from a positive pole to a negative pole.

___T___ 4. Capacitance, in electrical terms, is the ability of a device to store an electrical charge.

___F___ 5. Batteries generate alternating current.

___F___ 6. In physics, viscosity and density are basically the same thing.

___T___ 7. Boyle's law can be expressed as $P_1V_1 = P_2V_2$.

___F___ 8. According to Avogadro's law, each gram molecular weight of an ideal gas contains 5.9×10^{18} molecules.

___T___ 9. Graham's law states: $r = 1/\sqrt{D}$.

___F___ 10. Ionizing forms of radiation are never a threat to humans.

Multiple Choice

1. In science, a statement that describes a scientific proof is which of the following?

   a. theory
   b. hypothesis

   c. law
   d. principle

2. The MKSD system contains all of the following except:

   a. meter
   b. Kelvin

   c. second
   d. degree

3. 2,480,000 is the same as which of the following?

   a. 0.284×10^{-1}
   b. 2.84×10^{4}

   c. 2.84×10^{6}
   d. 2.84×10^{8}

4. Force is defined as which of the following?

   a. mass × acceleration
   b. distance ÷ time

   c. distance × velocity
   d. velocity × mass

5. Which of the following is a therapeutic modality affected by gravitational forces?

   a. oxygen therapy
   b. mechanical ventilation

   c. IPPB
   d. aerosol therapy

6. Which of the following devices functions to transform liquid to vapor?

   a. nebulizer
   b. humidifier

   c. ultrasonic
   d. ventilator

7. 100 mL of NaCl is dissolved in 3 L of water. What is the density of the NaCl?

   a. 33.3
   b. 300

   c. 3.33
   d. 0.033

8. If the pressure on one side of a tube is 90 mm Hg and the pressure on the other side is 45 mm Hg, what is the pressure gradient?

   a. 27
   b. 45

   c. 90
   d. 135

9. Which of the following are applications of the Venturi principle?

   1. jet nebulizer
   2. air entrainment mask
   3. nasal cannula
   4. nonrebreathing mask

   a. 1, 2
   b. 1, 3, 4

   c. 2, 3
   d. 3, 4

10. When measuring lung volumes, the gas being measured goes from body temperature to room temperature. The difference in temperature will cause inaccuracy unless the temperature is corrected. This is an application of which of the following?

    a. Charles's law
    b. Boyle's law

    c. Gay-Lussac's law
    d. Hooke's law

Lab Activities

1. Blow up a balloon, then release it to demonstrate the change from kinetic energy to potential energy. In what way does this resemble the action of individual alveoli?

2. It seems intuitive that if you drop two objects of different weight from a height, the heavier object will hit the ground first (Aristotle first proposed this; no scientist questioned it for 1500 years). Try an experiment in which you drop two similarly shaped objects of different weights (e.g., books) from a significant height (perhaps while standing on top of a desk—but be careful not to fall). What did you observe?

3. As a method for testing Poiseuille's law, try sucking water through a regular straw. Now try it through a coffee straw. What did you observe? You might also try the same experiment but replace the water with milk or even a milkshake. How is what you observed predicted by Poiseuille's law?

CHAPTER 4

Applied Chemistry

INTRODUCTION

In a living system, acids are substances that can donate electrons, and bases are substances that can receive electrons. The balance between acids and bases in body fluids, usually measured in terms of hydrogen ion concentration (pH), must be maintained for body systems to function.

Acids are categorized as strong or weak, depending on their degree of ionization. They are also further divided into bicarbonic (carbonic) and noncarbonic (fixed) acids. Fixed acids are eliminated daily by the kidneys, but carbonic acids can permeate cell membranes and affect cellular pH.

Buffers are substances that resist changes in pH when an acid or a base is added. Buffers are also divided into two broad categories: bicarbonate and nonbicarbonate. The bicarbonate–carbonic acid pair is the most important buffer in plasma. The nonbi-carbonate buffering systems include the phosphate, plasma protein, and hemoglobin buffer systems. Buffers are crucial for transporting carbon dioxide to the alveoli during respiration.

The body closely regulates the acid–base balance, but several factors can disturb it. Disturbances in the balance can be categorized as acidosis or alkalosis. Each can be further categorized according to its cause: respiratory or metabolic.

The respiratory system responds immediately to a change in the acid–base status and becomes maximal in 3–6 hours. In comparison, the renal response is slow and prolonged. The renal response is important because of its ability to conserve or increase acids or bases depending on whether the patient is in acidosis or alkalosis.

Discussion Activities and Questions

1. Using the periodic table, find the following:

   a. atomic number for oxygen

   b. symbol for carbon

   c. mass number for gold

2. Draw an oxygen atom.

3. Biological molecules are usually classified into which four groups?

4. Define and give an example of a polymer.

5. List three functions of proteins.

6. What is meant by "dissociation constant"?

7. Write the chemical reaction that results from the combination of CO_2 and H_2O.

8. What happens to the majority of CO_2 that diffuses into the blood from the cells?

9. Describe the six ways that CO_2 is carried in the blood.

10. According to the Henderson-Hasselbalch equation, pH = _____.

11. What is the purpose of carbonic anhydrase?

12. Describe the Haldane effect.

13. List three possible causes of respiratory acidosis.

14. Describe how the kidney works to compensate for a respiratory acidosis.

15. List the normal values for the following:

 a. pH

 b. PaO_2

 c. $PaCO_2$

 d. HCO_3

16. List three possible causes of metabolic acidosis.

REVIEW

True or False

—— 1. Protons are positively charged particles in the nucleus of an atom.

—— 2. The highest energy orbital in any atom is called an Is orbital.

—— 3. The atomic number of an atom is the sum of the protons and neutrons.

—— 4. In an atom, p orbitals have a dumbbell shape.

—— 5. Isotopes are atoms of the same element with different mass numbers.

_____ 6. Monosaccharides are not important energy sources.

_____ 7. Proteins are polymers consisting of amino acids.

_____ 8. Nucleic acids function to regulate metabolic activity in a cell.

_____ 9. Acids are substances that absorb or neutralize hydrogen ions.

_____ 10. A physiological buffer is a substance that resists changes in hydrogen ion concentration.

_____ 11. Acids are classified as strong or weak depending on their degree of ionization.

_____ 12. Respiration is a continuous interchange of oxygen and carbon dioxide.

Multiple Choice

1. Using the periodic table of the elements, which of the following is the atomic number for silver?

   a. 26
   b. 34
   c. 47
   d. 107

2. The nucleus of an atom contains which of the following atomic particles?

   1. quarks
   2. electrons
   3. neutrons
   4. protons

   a. 1, 3
   b. 1, 4
   c. 2, 3, 4
   d. 3, 4

3. Which type of bond is the result of sharing electrons between atoms?

   a. covalent
   b. ionic
   c. valent
   d. molecular

4. Carbohydrates can be subclassified into which of the following?

   a. fat
   b. protein
   c. lipid
   d. disaccharides

5. Naturally occurring proteins contain how many amino acids?

   a. 10
   b. 20
   c. 34
   d. 42

6. The Bronsted-Lowry concept defines acids as which of the following?

   a. neutron acceptors
   b. electron donors
   c. proton acceptors
   d. proton donors

7. The extracellular fluid compartment is subdivided into which of the following?

   1. cytoplasm
   2. plasma
   3. hemoglobin
   4. interstitial fluid

   a. 1, 2
   b. 1, 3, 4
   c. 2, 4
   d. 3, 4

8. Hydrogen ions are primarily produced from the formation of which of the following?

   a. gluconeogenesis
   b. carbon dioxide
   c. oxygen
   d. anaerobic metabolism

9. Following the dissociation of H_2CO_3 in the red blood cell, the HCO_3 that moves into the plasma does so in exchange for which of the following?

   a. Na

   b. K

   c. Ca

   d. Cl

10. A patient presents with severe hypoxia. This could result in which of the following acid–base states?

    a. metabolic alkalosis

    b. metabolic acidosis

    c. respiratory alkalosis

    d. respiratory acidosis

Lab Activity

1. Using a calculator with a log key, practice calculating pH, using various values for PCO_2 and HCO_3.

CHAPTER 5

Applied Microbiology

INTRODUCTION

Respiratory therapists work with many patients either who are susceptible to pulmonary infections or who have already developed pneumonia. An understanding of the types, identification, and management of pathogens capable of causing pulmonary disease can help practitioners minimize the occurrence and transmission of respiratory infections.

Organisms that can infect the lung include bacteria, viruses, fungi, and protozoa. Specific microorganisms are identified in the laboratory through a process that may use Gram staining, acid-fast testing, enzyme-linked immunosorbent assays, and cultures. Specimens may be obtained by having the patient cough, by suctioning, or by bronchoscopy. The specimens must be carefully collected and handled to avoid contamination and to provide accurate information.

Host defense mechanisms are the skin, the mucous membranes, and cellular and chemical responses to invasion. The immune response specifically generates protective antibodies in response to antigen challenges. Vaccines artificially stimulate antibody production to protect people from disease.

Disinfection and sterilization may be accomplished by means of physical methods, such as heat, pressure, radiation, sonic disruption, and filtration. The autoclave is an example of a device that incorporates both heat and pressure to sterilize medical items and equipment. Disinfection using the process of pasteurization is appropriate for many types of equipment used in respiratory care. Chemical agents may also be used for sterilization; ethylene oxide gas and gluteraldehyde solutions are two examples.

Antimicrobial drugs are key in the management of infections. However, because many pathogens have become drug-resistant as they mutate, the development of new agents is now of grave importance.

Infections may be transmitted by skin or mucous membrane contact, by airborne droplets, by contaminated food and water, by blood that has been contaminated by vectors, or by contact with contaminated inanimate objects. Thorough and frequent handwashing remains the most important procedure for limiting the transmission of infection.

Discussion Activities and Questions

1. Starting with the top, list the seven classification subdivisions.

2. Give two examples of a gram-negative bacillus.

3. What is ELISA?

4. List the six steps involved in all specimen collection.

5. What is susceptibility testing?

6. Describe opportunistic microorganisms and list two examples found in the human body.

7. Explain how having some resident microorganisms in the body can be beneficial.

8. Describe the two arms of the human immune system defenses.

9. List two parts of the body that are lined with mucous membranes. What would happen if the mucous membranes became dysfunctional?

10. What is the purpose of a fever?

11. List the five basic types of white blood cells and match them to their function.

12. Describe the body's response to a tissue injury. What are the visible manifestations of this response?

13. Discuss the various types of vaccines currently available, both for children and adults. Do you personally believe it is beneficial to get vaccinated against influenza?

14. Name a part of the body that provides an excellent environment for promoting microbial growth.

15. Explain the difference between disinfection and sterilization. List some common household disinfectants.

16. List four common methods of sterilization and give an example of an object that is best sterilized using each method.

17. What is meant by "virulence"?

18. List the four stages of the course of an infectious disease.

19. What is the difference between endemic and epidemic?

REVIEW

True or False

F   1. Viruses are included in the five-kingdom taxonomy.

T   2. The morphology of bacteria is easily observed under an ordinary light microscope.

F   3. Suctioning affords the best method for collecting sputum.

F   4. Microorganisms that are found in or on the body are referred to as *exogenous microflora*.

T   5. One of the effects of the inflammatory response is increased capillary permeability.

F   6. T-cells are named for the thyroid gland.

F   7. Asepsis and disinfection are the same thing.

F   8. A vector is an infectious microorganism.

T   9. Hospital instruments and equipment can be fomites.

T   10. *Streptococcus* is an important cause of pneumonia.

Multiple Choice

1. Which of the following bacterial characteristics provide information used for their classification and identification?

   1. morphology
   2. motility
   3. cytoplasm
   4. pathogenicity

   a. 1, 3
   b. 1, 2, 4
   c. 2, 3
   d. 3, 4

2. In Gram staining, a gram-positive microorganism would appear which color?

   a. white
   b. blue
   c. green
   d. purple

3. Which of the following sputum collection methods is best for obtaining anaerobic specimens and for cytology?

   a. bronchoscopy
   b. endotracheal suctioning
   c. nasotracheal suctioning
   d. coughing

4. Which of the following is one of the primary purposes for Gram staining and analyzing specimens for bacteria?

   a. to determine which specific antibiotic to administer
   b. to aid in the identification of bloodborne pathogens
   c. to aid in the diagnosis of pneumonia
   d. to determine which respiratory therapy modalities will be effective

5. Which of the following is not included in the innate arm of the immune system defenses?

   a. mechanical barriers
   b. complement
   c. phagocytes
   d. IgG antibodies

6. Injured cells release which of the following chemicals, triggering the inflammatory response?

   1. complement
   2. prostaglandin
   3. histamine
   4. bradykinin

   a. 1, 2
   b. 1, 3, 4
   c. 2, 3
   d. 3, 4

7. A patient presents to the ER in shock secondary to a bee sting. Which of the following immunoglobulins most likely caused the problem?

   a. IgA
   b. IgD
   c. IgE
   d. IgM

8. Which of the following would be the best method of cleaning your stethoscope after using it on a patient?

   a. soak in gluteraldehyde
   b. expose to ethylene oxide
   c. cleanse with isopropyl alcohol
   d. pasteurize

9. Which of the following is recommended for disinfecting home equipment?

   a. white vinegar
   b. isopropyl alcohol
   c. phenol solution
   d. bleach

10. You are seeing a patient with HIV who has been diagnosed with *Pneumocystis* pneumonia. Which of the following antimicrobials might you administer?

    a. pentamidine
    b. tobramycin
    c. ribavirin
    d. vancomycin

Matching

Match the immunoglobulins to their functions.

_e_ 1. IgA

_d_ 2. IgD

_b_ 3. IgE

_a_ 4. IgG

_c_ 5. IgM

a. secondary immune response

b. causes allergic responses

c. primary immune response

d. controls stimulation of B-cells

e. protects the mucous membranes

Lab Activities

1. Look around the respiratory therapy lab. How would you sterilize or disinfect some of the items?

2. Discuss what methods of sterilization and/or disinfection the respiratory care departments in your area use.

3. Have you ever had to take antibiotics? If so, what was the specific drug and why was it prescribed?

4. Have you ever had an infectious disease (e.g., flu, pneumonia, etc.)? If so, describe the stages your body went through.

Cardiopulmonary Anatomy and Physiology

INTRODUCTION

The cardiopulmonary system brings atmospheric gas into the lungs, through successively smaller airways, to the alveoli. In the alveoli, these gases are brought into close contact with pulmonary capillary blood from the pulmonary vascular system, and oxygen rapidly moves into the blood and carbon dioxide out of it.

Breathing and circulation are controlled efficiently, balancing benefit and energy expenditure to meet the body's always-changing needs. General science principles clarify lung ventilation, gas diffusion, the perfusion of blood, gas transportation, and cellular delivery mechanisms.

The fetus and newborn have different lung function and circulatory patterns than adults. Aging, exercise, and high-altitude and high-pressure environments all affect respiratory function.

Discussion Activities and Questions

1. Describe the purpose of the Valsalva maneuver.

2. Describe the structure and function of the mucociliary system:

    a. How can this system be damaged by disease?

    b. What would be the consequences if it is damaged?

c. How can the respiratory therapist assist in the removal of mucus?

3. Describe what happens to the airways during an asthma attack. What would be an effective way to treat this?

4. Describe the function of surfactant. What would be the consequences if surfactant production was decreased or absent?

5. Describe the autonomic nervous system.

6. During the insertion of an endotracheal tube, if the tube is pushed down too far (past the carina), it is much more likely to enter the right mainstem bronchus. Why?

7. Describe the relationship between the visceral pleura and parietal pleura. What would be the consequences if this relationship were damaged?

8. What factors will increase or decrease airway resistance?

9. Using the concept of time constants, explain how inhaled gas will be distributed if one lung has a higher airway resistance than the other.

10. What is dead space ventilation? How is the amount of anatomic dead space determined?

11. Explain what happens to the ventilatory pattern when lung compliance is decreased.

12. Explain the difference between tachypnea, hyperpnea, and dyspnea.

13. Explain why the wall of the left ventricle is thicker than the wall of the right ventricle.

14. Explain the differences between the pulmonary and systemic circulations.

15. Describe the three factors that determine ventricular preload.

16. Describe the Bohr effect.

17. What is the significance of $C_{A-v}O_2$?

18. List three causes of shunting.

19. Describe how the kidney works to compensate for a respiratory alkalosis or acidosis.

20. Describe how a ventilation/perfusion ratio is determined.

21. Describe the difference between the respiratory quotient and the respiratory exchange ratio.

22. Describe how the central chemoreceptor regulates breathing.

23. Explain why respiratory therapists must carefully monitor and control oxygen therapy in patients with chronic hypercapnia (high carbon dioxide levels).

24. Describe fetal circulation.

25. List three ways your body may adapt to higher elevations.

REVIEW

True or False

_____ 1. The vibrissae are located in the bronchi.

_____ 2. The soft palate closes the opening between the nasopharynx and the oropharynx.

_____ 3. The regulatory zone ends at generation 23.

_____ 4. Increased parasympathetic activity increases mucus production.

_____ 5. Clara cells are important in providing collateral circulation.

_____ 6. Type II alveolar cells produce macrophages.

_____ 7. Arteries always carry oxygenated blood.

_____ 8. The right lung is larger, heavier, and shorter than the left.

_____ 9. The chest wall's natural tendency is to recoil.

_____ 10. The transpulmonary pressure is the difference between alveolar pressure and pleural pressure.

_____ 11. Atelectasis is the collapse of small alveoli.

_____ 12. When airway resistance increases, ventilatory rate and tidal volume usually increase.

_____ 13. Serum is plasma without the factors involved in clotting.

_____ 14. Transmural pressure is the difference between intravascular pressure and the pressure external to that vessel.

_____ 15. The majority of pulmonary blood flow is distributed to the apices.

_____ 16. According to the oxyhemoglobin dissociation curve, increasing a patient's PaO_2 from 80 to 100 mm Hg will result in a significant increase in SaO_2.

_____ 17. Hypoxia is defined as a low oxygen concentration in the arterial blood.

_____ 18. The body compensates for respiratory acidosis by excreting bicarbonate through the kidney.

_____ 19. The Hering-Breuer reflex serves to trigger expiration.

_____ 20. A baby breathes in utero.

_____ 21. As a person ages, residual volume tends to decrease.

_____ 22. During exercise, $PaCO_2$ remains constant.

Multiple Choice

1. The bronchial blood supply is about what percent of the cardiac output?

   a. 1
   b. 5

   c. 8
   d. 12

2. Bronchodilation can be facilitated by stimulating which of the following receptors?

   a. beta 2
   b. alpha

   c. gamma
   d. beta 1

3. A young male is involved in a diving accident that severs the spinal cord at the level of the fifth cervical vertebra. Which of the following would be the pulmonary consequences?

   a. Ventilation would be normal
   b. The diaphragm would cease to contract
   c. Ventilation would be normal, but the patient would not be able to cough
   d. All ventilation would cease

4. To generate an effective cough, which of the following muscles should be active?

   a. external intercostals
   b. pectoralis major
   c. sternocleidomastoid
   d. rectus abdominus

5. Based on the following data, the static lung compliance is which of the following (in mL/cm H_2O)?

Volume	600 mL
Rate	12 bpm
Pressure	20 cm H_2O

   a. 15
   b. 30
   c. 50
   d. 240

6. Based on the following data, what is the airway resistance (in cm H_2O/L/sec)?

Volume	0.5 L
Transairway pressure	5 cm H_2O
Flow	0.5 L/sec

   a. 1
   b. 5
   c. 10
   d. 20

7. Based on the following data, what is the V_E?

   | Rate | 16 bpm |
   | Volume | 600 mL |

   a. 5.4 L
   b. 6.1 L
   c. 8.1 L
   d. 9.6 L

8. A person experiences an acute exacerbation of COPD, which causes him to trap air (air trapping). Which of the following is most likely to increase as a consequence?

   a. expiratory reserve volume
   b. residual volume
   c. vital capacity
   d. tidal volume

9. Based on the following data, what is the alveolar PO_2 (P_AO_2) in mm Hg?

P_B	720 mm Hg
F_IO_2	0.4
Rate	16 bpm

   a. 155
   b. 193
   c. 269
   d. 285

10. Which of the following will cause a decrease in the diffusion of oxygen across the alveolar-capillary membrane?

    a. increased P_AO_2
    b. decreased alveolar surface area
    c. decreased alveolar-capillary thickness
    d. increased ventilatory rate

11. You are seeing a patient who has become dehydrated. Which of the following will be directly affected?

    a. heart rate
    b. afterload
    c. diastolic pressure
    d. preload

12. Which of the following is an active mechanism that affects vascular resistance?

    a. increased PCO_2
    b. increased pH

    c. lung volume changes
    d. increased P_AO_2

13. A person presents to the ER because of exposure to carbon monoxide. The patient is most likely experiencing which of the following?

    a. anemic hypoxia
    b. hypoxic hypoxia

    c. circulatory hypoxia
    d. histotoxic hypoxia

14. Which of the following is the best interpretation of the following data?

    pH   7.28
    $PaCO_2$ 55 mm Hg
    HCO_3 25 mEq

    a. respiratory acidosis
    b. respiratory alkalosis

    c. metabolic acidosis
    d. metabolic alkalosis

Matching

Match the response with the specific component of the autonomic nervous system:

_____ 1. pupil dilation
_____ 2. bronchoconstriction
_____ 3. bradycardia
_____ 4. hypertension
_____ 5. increased intestinal peristalsis

a. parasympathetic
b. sympathetic

Match the hemodynamic value with its corresponding normal range:

_____ 6. cardiac output
_____ 7. pulmonary capillary wedge pressure
_____ 8. central venous pressure
_____ 9. mean pulmonary arterial pressure

a. 0–8 mm Hg
b. 4–8 Lpm
c. 9–18 mm Hg
d. 4–12 mm Hg

Lab Activities

1. Using a tongue depressor and a dental mirror, examine the oropharynx of a lab partner.

2. Using a laryngoscope, examine the structures in the laryngopharynx of an intubation mannequin.

3. Blow up a new balloon (no fair stretching it first!). At what point was it hardest to inflate? Draw a rough graph of the compliance of the balloon. What does the graph resemble?

4. Using a ventilator and a double lung simulator, observe the effect on distribution of ventilation when you have different airway resistance and/or compliance in one of the lungs.

5. Measure the pulse and respiratory rate of a partner at rest. Now have your partner engage in aerobic exercise (e.g., running in place, going up several flights of stairs). Remeasure the pulse and respiratory rate immediately upon conclusion of the exercise. What did you observe? Why?

CHAPTER 7

Cardiopulmonary Pharmacology

INTRODUCTION

A working knowledge of key pharmacological terms and concepts, as well as the dosages, actions, contraindications, and side effects of the major pharmaceutical agents, is critical to the practicing respiratory therapist in any area of patient care. Whether the practitioner is administering medicated aerosol treatments, providing conscious sedation during certain diagnostic and therapeutic procedures under medical supervision, or reviewing medications with a patient, this knowledge makes the respiratory therapist more clinically competent.

Discussion Activities and Questions

1. What are some methods of delivering bronchodilators to mechanically ventilated patients, as recommended by clinical practice guidelines?

   Large volume neb, ultrasonic nebs, small volume nebs, metered dose inhalers

2. If an asthmatic uses multiple MDIs, what should the general sequence be?

   Bronchodialator, mast cell inhibitor, corticosteroid

3. What are some side effects associated with inhaled bronchodilators?

REVIEW

Multiple Choice

1. What is the term for the time required for drug absorption, drug action, drug distribution in the body, and destabilization and excretion of the drug?

   a. pharmacokinetic phase
   b. pharmaceutical phase
   c. pharmacodynamic phase
   d. both a and b

2. What is the term for when increased amounts of a drug are needed to produce the desired effect?

   a. tachyphylaxis
   b. tolerance
   c. therapeutic index (TI)
   d. both a and b

3. What is the term for when two or more drugs produce an effect or response that neither could produce alone?

   a. therapeutic index (TI)
   b. additive effect
   c. synergy
   d. both a and b

4. Which of the following are drugs that work by disrupting the mucus molecule?

   a. anticholinergic
   b. wetting agents
   c. antimicrobials
   d. mucolytics

5. What is the term for when two drugs have the opposite effect?

   a. therapeutic index (TI)
   b. antagonism
   c. additive effect
   d. both a and b

6. Drugs that promote bronchodilation via the neurotransmitter norepinehrine are:

   a. adrenergic
   b. anticholinergic
   c. mucolytic
   d. antimicrobial

Matching

Match these terms with their definitions on the right.

_C_ 1. Surfactant

_d_ 2. Ethyl alcohol

_a_ 3. Pharmacology

a. the study of drugs

b. how a drug is delivered to the body

c. used in treating IRDS

b 4. Pharmaceutical phase

f 5. Sympathomimetic bronchodilator

g 6. Anticholinergic

e 7. Acetylcysteine

d. used to treat pulmonary edema

e. a mucolytic

f. also called adrenergic

g. also referred to as parasympatholytics

Lab Activities

1. In small groups, use flash cards to familiarize students with the generic and brand names of common respiratory drugs. Also discuss the indications for using these drugs, along with contraindications and side effects.

2. In a large-group setting, introduce different case scenarios and ask the group for feedback on which type of drug would be appropriate in each scenario, as well as contraindications and side effects.

Case Studies

1. A 45-year-old patient presents to the Emergency Room in moderate respiratory distress. His vital signs are heart rate 98 bpm, respiratory rate 38 bpm, room air pulse ox 90%, temp 37 Celsius. He speaks in short sentences and explains that he was playing baseball at a family picnic when he started experiencing shortness of breath. He has a past medical history of asthma and normally uses an Advair inhaler for maintenance. He states that he lost his job recently and has not been able to afford the inhaler, so he has not used it in two months. Based on this information, what type of bronchodilator would you recommend for this patient and why?

   albuterol b/c it is a rescue inhaler

2. While doing AM rounds at the hospital, one of the patients who was admitted for asthma exacerbation is being discharged to home. The patient is uncertain which medication that has been prescribed is the rescue medication and which is the controller medication. The medications that have been prescribed for home use are Flovent and Combivent. Which would you identify as the rescue medication? Which is the controller medication?

CHAPTER 8

Pulmonary Infections

INTRODUCTION

Infections of the respiratory tract are among the most common infections of the human race. In the United States, respiratory tract infections are responsible for more visits to physicians than any other diseases and for more time lost from work or school.

Viruses, bacteria, fungi, and parasites are organisms that cause infections of the respiratory system. Some of these infections are contagious and may cause serious respiratory disease.

Pneumonia, an infection of one or both lungs, is extremely contagious and is the result of breathing in small droplets that get into the air when an infected person coughs or sneezes. Pneumonia can also result when bacteria or viruses from the mouth, throat, or nose inadvertently enter the lungs.

Antibiotics are used to treat pneumonia caused by bacteria, the most common cause of the condition. Pneumonia can also be caused by viruses, such as those that cause influenza (flu) and chickenpox (varicella). Varicella pneumonia, which is rare, can be treated with antiviral medicine.

In most cases pneumonia is a short-term, treatable illness. But frequent bouts of pneumonia can be a serious complication of a long-term (chronic) illness, such as chronic obstructive pulmonary disease (COPD).

M. tuberculosis infection is transmissible from person to person by way of inhalation of organisms suspended in aerosolized drops of saliva, respiratory tract secretions, or other body fluids. If the organisms are able to multiply in the lung, they can spread there and into other organs. Any patient with an evaluation suggestive of active tuberculosis should be placed in respiratory isolation.

Two patient populations at high risk of pulmonary infections are the elderly and patients who are immunocompromised. In these groups, the mortality rate from pulmonary infections can be very high. To implement an effective treatment plan, the respiratory therapist should know the signs and symptoms of infection and get a comprehensive patient history. Health-care workers who may be exposed to pneumonia should also know the signs and symptoms, as well as infection control precautions.

Discussion Activities and Questions

1. Describe the difference between tuberculosis exposure and tuberculosis infection.

2. List some fungal infections and the geographical areas they may be found in.

3. What are some differences between bacterial and viral infections?

Thought Question

1. TB is closely associated with HIV. List some ways that could help bring better awareness to HIV patients and other immunicompromised patients who are at risk of contracting TB.

REVIEW

Multiple Choice

1. A cheese-like material seen in some granulomas is called:

   a. Ghon complex
   b. Ranke complex

   c. lymphokines
   d. caseous necrosis

2. Up to 50% of HIV-positive individuals will develop this before their death:

   a. mycobacterium avian complex
   b. COPD

   c. Legionnaire's disease
   d. pulmonary hypertension

3. Nephrotoxicity is a possible complication of which of the following drugs?

   a. isoniazid
   b. amphoterin B

   c. rifampin
   d. albuterol

4. This stage of lobar pneumonia occurs 4–5 days postinfection and is characterized by alveoli containing many polymorph nuclear leukocytes and very few red blood cells.

   a. inflammatory stage
   b. gray hepatization stage
   c. red hepatization stage
   d. resolution stage

5. *Legionella pneumophilia* can often be found where?

   a. Ohio River valley
   b. western Canada
   c. southeastern United States
   d. stagnant water reservoirs

6. A term used to describe a tuberculous lesion that erodes into a blood vessel and allows organisms to spread throughout the body is:

   a. miliary tuberculosis
   b. Ranke complex
   c. Ghon complex
   d. granuloma

7. What is the name for the test in which tuberculin protein is injected intradermally?

   a. Mantoux test
   b. bronchoalveolar lavage
   c. Brachey therapy
   d. acid-fast smear

8. Risk factors for community-acquired pneumonia include:

   a. alcoholism
   b. smoking
   c. poor nutrition
   d. older age
   e. a, c, and d
   f. a, b, and d
   g. all of the above

Matching

Match these terms with their definitions on the right.

_____ 1. polymicrobial

_____ 2. anergic

_____ 3. mycelium

_____ 4. bullae

a. diminished hypersensitivity

b. enlarged alveoli

c. long, branching filamentous tubes

d. more than one species

Airflow Limitation Diseases

INTRODUCTION

The airflow limitation diseases discussed in this chapter are asthma, chronic bronchitis, bronchiectasis, and emphysema. Asthma is in a separate category of airflow limitation because it is a reversible disease that responds to bronchodilator therapy. Chronic bronchitis, bronchiectasis, and emphysema are known by the acronym COPD. The airway obstruction in these diseases is not reversed by bronchodilators, and the disease results in permanent and progressive changes. In people who are asthmatic, the inflammation causes recurrent episodes of wheezing, dyspnea, chest tightness, and coughing. The airflow obstruction may reverse spontaneously, or it may require treatment for reversal. Exposure to environmental triggers elicits a hypersensitivity reaction in the bronchial epithelium of allergic patients, which may result in a rapid worsening in respiratory function. Other causes of exacerbation are viral infection, exercise, and inhalation of irritants.

COPD is characterized by the presence of chronic bronchitis, emphysema, or both. The COPD patient has progressive airflow limitation that may be partially reversible in those patients with hyper-reactive airways. Emphysema is present when there are permanent dilation and destruction of lung units distal to the terminal bronchioles.

Chronic bronchitis is the predominant cause of COPD. Chronic bronchitis is defined functionally as an individual having a chronically productive cough lasting 3 or more consecutive months for 2 successive years. Bronchiectasis is an anatomic distortion of the conducting airways that results in chronic cough, sputum production, and recurrent cough. The airway dilation is chronic and irreversible, usually affecting medium-sized airways. It is the result of recurring episodes of infection and inflammation.

A deficiency of alph-1 antitrypsin is a genetic disease involving a decreased ability to block the activity of proteolytic enzymes. A deficiency in the enzyme results in the unopposed proteolysis of elastin in the lung and the liver. The increased breakdown of elastin leads to the development of panacinar emphysema.

Basic spirometry is the gold standard for diagnosing airflow limitation. Forced expiratory maneuvers identify airflow limitation and its severity. The differentiation between emphysema and other diseases that limit airflow is based on the measurement of carbon monoxide diffusing capacity. Because emphysema results in the loss of alveolar surface area, the carbon monoxide diffusing capacity of the lung is decreased.

The major complications of COPD are frequent infections, cor pulmonale, respiratory failure, sleeping disorders, and pneumothorax. These complications can cause deterioration of the patient's quality and length of life.

Discussion Activities and Questions

1. What are some etiological factors associated with asthma and emphysema?

2. List some of the changes during the three phases of airway inflammation.

3. List some of the causes of bronchiectasis.

Thought Questions

1. In an acute asthma attack, what medications would you select for treatment and why?

2. As discussed in the chapter, many of these diseases have overlapping signs and symptoms. What areas on a patient history and assessment could help you determine if a patient has asthma or COPD?

REVIEW

Multiple Choice

1. This pulmonary function study helps determine the difference between emphysema and other COPD diseases:

    a. peak flow
    b. forced vital capacity

    c. diffusion study
    d. minute volume

2. The most general criterion for COPD is:

    a. FEV1/FVC < 70
    b. FEV1/FVC > 70

    c. PEFR 80% of predicted
    d. PEFR > 75% of predicted

3. A chronic cough of mucopurulent secretions is associated with:

    a. asthma
    b. COPD

    c. bronchitis
    d. bronchiectasis

4. Which of the following could trigger asthma symptoms?

    a. exercise
    b. aspirin
    c. cold air
    d. foods containing sulfites

    e. a and b
    f. a, b, and d
    g. all of the above

5. The most effective drugs for long-term asthma maintenance are:

    a. short-acting beta-2 bronchodilators
    b. corticosteroids
    c. long-acting beta-2 agonists
    d. anticholinergics

    e. a and c
    f. b and c
    g. c and d

Matching

Match these terms with their definitions on the right.

_____ 1. Atopy

_____ 2. Vagal tone

_____ 3. Centriacinar emphysema

_____ 4. Paraseptal emphysema

_____ 5. Cor pulmonale

a. occurs in upper lungs, associated with smoking

b. exposure to an antigen to which a person is sensitive

c. commonly occurs in lung apices

d. right heart failure

e   hyperexcitability of parasympathetic nervous system

Lab Activity

1. In the lab, demonstrate how to perform bedside spirometry tests using the handheld machine. The students can be familiarized with values indicating COPD or asthma.

CHAPTER 10

Diffuse Parenchymal Lung Diseases

INTRODUCTION

Diffuse parenchymal diseases encompass all of the pulmonary and systemic diseases that cause infiltration into the alveolar airspace and interstitium of the lung. The infiltration results in the thickening of the alveolar capillary membrane with an associated decrease in lung compliance and gas exchange. The wide variety of diseases that cause diffuse parenchymal and interstitial damage range, among many others, from idiopathic lung diseases, environmental lung diseases, drug toxicity, and collagen vascular diseases to hemorrhagic diseases of the lung.

Many of the DPLDs have an unknown etiology. However, of the diseases having known etiologies, a large group of diseases consists of the environmental (occupational) lung diseases. Environmental lung diseases are the most common disease classification of all the DPLDs. These diseases are distributed geographically according to the industry and occupational concentrations in specific areas of the country.

Fibrosis is the result of chronic inflammation due to persistent or recurrent exposure to a stimulant, irritant, or antigen causing parenchymal injury.

The major clinical manifestation of people with interstitial lung disease is dyspnea. It is usually gradual in onset, with the patient believing that he or she is just "out of shape" until the dyspnea progresses ultimately to dyspnea at rest.

All forms of DPLD decrease lung volumes but preserve expiratory flow rates unless the patient has airway involvement, is a smoker, or has an airflow limitation lung disease. The patients have a reduced total lung capacity, vital capacity, functional residual capacity, and FEV1, along with a normal or increased FEV1/FVC ratio. Studies of gas transfer typically show a reduction of carbon monoxide–diffusing capacity. The primary reason for the reduced diffusion is the destruction of alveoli and their capillaries, decreasing available surface area for gas exchange.

The major complications of DPLD are cor pulmonale, exacerbation of idiopathic pulmonary fibrosis, and progressive oxygenation failure. These complications can cause a significant decrease in quality and length of life.

Treatment of DPLD varies with the underlying disease, but the general treatment has not changed in years. The initial direction in treatment is to control exposure to the precipitating antigens. Because many diseases causing DPLD do not have a known etiology, this measure is effective only in cases of environmental exposure.

The drug treatment used for people with DPLD is to prevent disease progression by suppressing the inflammatory process in the lung. This goal is accomplished by administering high-dose corticosteroids and monitoring disease activity by chest radiograph, HRCT, or other techniques. If steroids effectively reduce inflammation, the patient's dose is tapered to a level where inflammation suppression is sustained; this daily dose is maintained for long-term administration. Other drugs that may be used are cytotoxic drugs such as cyclophosphamide or azathioprine.

Continuous oxygen therapy is another treatment option that is predominately supportive. Continuous oxygen therapy may support the patient's oxygenation temporarily, but disease progression causes hypoxemia that is increasingly unresponsive to oxygen. Without a lung transplant, the patient will die when the disease process is so extensive that oxygenation cannot be maintained with supplemental oxygen. Lung transplantation is a definitive treatment for the patient with DPLD. Ideally, there should be early referral for lung transplantation.

Discussion Activities and Questions

1. List the four types of idiopathic interstitial pneumonias.

2. What are some occupations associated with the incidence of silicosis?

3. What pulmonary function values are you likely to see in patients with DPLD?

REVIEW

Multiple Choice

1. Which PFT finding is consistent in patients with DPLD?

   a. increased TLC
   b. decreased DLCO
   c. increased PEFR
   d. increased FEV/FVC ratio

2. Honeycomb lung is often used to describe:

   a. granuloma formation
   b. enlarged alveoli
   c. severe pulmonary fibrosis
   d. enlarged lymph nodes

3. Factors that affect the survival rates for people with interstitial pulmonary fibrosis include:

   a. X-ray changes
   b. gender
   c. age
   d. race

4. Which of the following statements concerning environmental lung diseases are true?

   a. Pollutant particle density plays a part in development of environmental lung disease.
   b. It is the most common disease classification of the different types of DPLD.
   c. They occur mainly in the southern United States.
   d. Most have no known etiology.

e. a and c

f. a and b

g. all of the above

5.   The definitive treatment for DPLD is:

a. lung transplant

b. oxygen therapy

c. corticosteroids

d. bronchodilators

6.   This toxic gas is found in pesticide and rubber production:

a. ammonia

b. chloramine

c. methyl isocyanate

d. chlorine

7.   This disease has a higher degree of incidence in African Americans:

a. sarcoidosis

b. silicosis

c. asbestosis

d. Goodpastures syndrome

8.   *Aspergillus clavatus* is one of the known antigens of this disease:

a. silicosis

b. malt workers lung

c. sarcoidosis

d. asbestosis

Matching

Match these terms with their definitions on the right.

_____ 1. exacerbation

_____ 2. cor pulmonale

_____ 3. fibrosis

_____ 4. etiology

_____ 5. pathogenesis

a. cause

b. evolution

c. worsening

d. right heart failure

e. thickening

Case Study

1.   Mr. Jones is a 47-year-old man who has worked in a coal mine since the age of 18. He presents to the doctor's office with a complaint of increasing shortness of breath, especially on exertion. In addition to a physical exam and patient history, what other tests could you recommend to help rule out the presence of DPLD?

CHAPTER 11

Atelectasis, Pleural Disorders, and Lung Cancer

INTRODUCTION

Atelectasis is the incomplete expansion of the lung. It can be categorized in several ways, but the simplest is dividing it into obstructive, nonobstructive, and special types of lung collapse. *Obstructive atelectasis,* the most common type, results from the reabsorption of gas from the lung distal to the obstruction. *Nonobstructive* types of atelectasis are caused by an abnormal relationship between the visceral and parietal pleura, a loss of surfactant, or the replacement of normal lung parenchyma with scar tissue or cellular infiltrates. One of the common *special* types of atelectasis is acute atelectasis after surgery, especially procedures involving the thorax or upper abdomen, which has long been associated with the loss of lung volume, causing complete or partial alveolar collapse. Pain, medications, increased secretions, and the inability to cough and to take deep breaths are common causes of postoperative atelectasis. The treatment of atelectasis depends on the underlying cause. The goal of treatment is lung reinflation by removing the cause of the lung collapse.

Pleural disorders are pleural abnormalities that develop because of another primary disease or disorder. The pleural surface may become inflamed or irritated, or the pleural space may be filled with air, gas, or fluid. Pneumothorax is the presence of free air in the pleural space that causes partial or complete collapse of the affected lung. Pleural effusions are an accumulation of fluid in the pleural space. The most common cause of pleural effusion is congestive heart failure (30–40% of cases). The remaining 60–70% of the cases of pleural effusion are divided among nine primary diseases, with pneumonia as the second most common cause and malignancy as the third.

The two major classifications of lung cancer are non-small-cell lung cancer (NSCLC) and small-cell lung cancer (SCLC). NSCLC accounts for approximately 75% of all lung cancers, and it is a heterogeneous collection of three histological cell types: adenocarcinoma, squamous-cell carcinoma, and large-cell carcinoma. These histologies are classified together because the approaches to diagnosis, staging/prognosis, and treatment are similar. Small-cell lung cancer is very different from the other cancer classification with a different staging process, treatment approach, and prognosis.

The treatment of lung cancer depends on the cell type: non-small-cell lung cancer or small-cell lung cancer. The sensitivity of the tumors to radiation, chemotherapy, and the ability to surgically remove the tumor all vary in these two cancer classifications.

Discussion Activities and Questions

1. What are some risk factors associated with lung cancer?

2. What are some clinical findings associated with atelectasis?

3. What are some clinical findings associated with a pneumothorax?

REVIEW

Multiple Choice

1. Tracheal deviation to the affected side characterizes:

   a. pneumothorax
   b. atelectasis

   c. lung cancer
   d. asthma

2. Primary spontaneous pneumothorax mainly occurs in:

   a. African Americans
   b. male smokers between the ages of 20 and 40

   c. endomorphic females
   d. the elderly population

3. An empyema is:

   a. fluid in the lung
   b. pus in the lung

   c. air in the lung
   d. a foreign body in the lung

4. The most important risk factor for lung cancer is:

   a. hormonal influences
   b. air pollution

   c. occupation
   d. cigarette smoking

5. The most common cause of plural effusions is:

   a. congestive heart failure
   b. lung cancer

   c. asthma
   d. infection

6. The primary treatment for non-small-cell lung cancer is:

   a. radiation
   b. surgery
   c. decortication
   d. thoracentesis

   e. a and d
   f. a and b
   g. c and d

7. Extracting fluid by use of a needle is:

   a. bronchoscopy
   b. brachytherapy

   c. thoracentesis
   d. chemotherapy

Matching

Match these terms with their definitions on the right.

_____ 1. Transudate

_____ 2. Pleural effusion

_____ 3. Thoracentesis

_____ 4. Atelectasis

_____ 5. Empyema

a. has high concentration of protein

b. has low concentration of protein

c. incomplete expansion of lung

d. inserting needle into pleural space

e. pus in pleural space

f. fluid in pleural space

Lab Activity

1. In the lab in various stations, items associated with the disorders discussed in this chapter can be displayed for the students to examine. Recommended items include chest tube kits, samples of syringes used for thoracentesis, and X-ray images. The instructor might assign a hands-on activity in which students perform a simulated assessment and give feedback as to what clinical signs associated with the various pleural disorders would be present. In addition, printed supplemental materials concerning lung cancer, types of lung cancer, and treatment options could be made available to students as well.

Case Study

1. A 27-year-old man presents to the Emergency Room in moderate respiratory distress. The patient states that he began to feel short of breath after shoveling snow. His vital signs are: heart rate, 112 bpm; respiratory rate, 32 bpm; temp, 37°C; SpO$_2$ on room air, 94%; breath sounds clear on left but almost absent on right side. The patient has no significant past medical history; he does not drink but he does smoke two packs of cigarettes a day.

   a. Based on these findings, what would you suspect is the cause of this patient's symptoms?

   b. What might you see on this person's chest X-ray?

   c. What would be a treatment option for this patient?

CHAPTER 12

Diseases That Affect the Pulmonary Vasculature

INTRODUCTION

Pulmonary edema is a condition caused by excess fluid in the lungs. This fluid collects in the interstitial spaces and may enter the alveolar space, interfering with ventilation and gas exchange. In most cases, cardiac problems cause pulmonary edema. Fluid can accumulate for other reasons, including pneumonia, exposure to certain toxins and medications, exercising, or living at high elevations and malnutrition. Treatment for pulmonary edema varies depending on the cause, but generally includes supplemental oxygen and medications.

Cardiogenic pulmonary edema—also known as congestive heart failure—occurs when the diseased or overworked left ventricle cannot effectively pump out the blood it receives from the lungs. As a result, pressure increases inside the left atrium and then in the pulmonary veins and capillaries, causing fluid to be pushed through the capillary walls into the interstitial spaces and alveoli.

If not treated, pulmonary edema can raise pressure in the pulmonary artery, and eventually the right ventricle will begin to fail. The increased pressure backs up into the right atrium and then into various parts of the body. When not treated, acute pulmonary edema can be fatal. In some instances it may be fatal even if the patient receives treatment. Oxygen administration is the first step in treatment for pulmonary edema. It may be necessary to assist ventilation mechanically.

Diseases of the lung can cause right heart disease and subsequently right heart failure (cor pulmonale). Although other conditions can cause hypertrophy of the right ventricle associated with cor pulmonale, very often it is caused by chronic obstructive pulmonary disease.

Embolization of the pulmonary vasculature is generally the result of blood clots (thrombi) in the lower extremities. When emboli form in the lungs, they block venous circulation to distal alveoli, resulting in dead space ventilation. Obstruction of the pulmonary vascular bed greater than 50% can be catastrophic. The goals of treatment for pulmonary embolism are to maintain oxygenation, and prevent new thrombus formation and further extension of the embolus until fibrinolysis can occur.

In ARDS, structural changes occur: alveolar and interstitial edema, alveolar consolidation, loss of pulmonary surfactant, and atelectasis. The general management of ARDS requires modalities such as oxygen therapy, mechanical ventilation using a lung protective strategy, and techniques to reinflate collapsed alveoli.

Discussion Activities and Questions

1. What are some diseases associated with cor pulmonale?

2. What are some drugs that may be used to treat cardiogenic pulmonary edema?

3. List the clinical criteria required for the diagnosis of ARDS.

REVIEW

Multiple Choice

1. ARDS is commonly associated with:

   a. long plane rides
   b. right heart failure
   c. injury to alveolar capillary interface
   d. history of smoking

2. Inspiratory rales are often heard in patients with:

   a. pulmonary edema
   b. sarcoidosis
   c. pulmonary embolus
   d. kyphoscoliosis

3. High ventilating or PEEP pressures may cause:

   a. pulmonary embolus
   b. barotrauma
   c. Homan's sign
   d. Kerley's lines

4. A pulmonary capillary wedge pressure of <18 mm HG is often detected in patients with:

   a. asthma
   b. sleep apnea
   c. sarcoidosis
   d. ARDS

5. The anticoagulant of choice to treat a pulmonary embolus is:

   a. dobutamine
   b. heparin
   c. furosemide
   d. albuterol

6. Ankle and leg edema, distended neck veins, and pulsus alternans are signs associated with:

   a. pulmonary edema
   b. sleep apnea
   c. ARDS
   d. pulmonary embolus

Matching

Match these terms with their definitions on the right.

_____ 1. loop diuretics

_____ 2. cor pulmonale

_____ 3. Homan's sign

_____ 4. barotrauma

_____ 5. Kerley's lines

a. calf pain

b. right heart failure

c. chest wall deformity

d. detected on X-ray of patient with pulmonary edema

e. used to treat pulmonary edema

f. caused by high PEEP pressures

Case Study

1. An 84-year-old man presents to the Emergency Department in moderate to severe respiratory distress. His vital signs are: heart rate, 122 bpm; respiratory rate, 34 bpm; blood pressure, 175/95; temp, 37.5°C; breath sounds, inspiratory rales throughout all lung fields; pulse ox on room air, 85%. You observe dependent edema in the patient's legs.

   a.   Based on these symptoms, what is this patient experiencing?

   After applying oxygen, the patient is still severely short of breath and his pulse ox on a 50% Venti-mask is 89%. Arterial blood gasses drawn on this FIO_2 are PH. 7.41, PCO_2 57, PO_2 54.
   The emergency physician has ordered a loop diuretic, but is concerned that the patient may need to be intubated.

   b.   What can you recommend to the physician that might both aid the patient until the diuretic begins to work and possibly avoid intubation?

Essential Diagnostics

Comprehensive History, Assessment, and Documentation

INTRODUCTION

A health-care professional must act like a detective to determine what is wrong with a patient. Thorough questioning and an in-depth examination of the patient should reveal any medical problems. In most cases, an extensive history and physical exam decreases the need for invasive testing and accurately indicates what tests are necessary. Also, as respiratory therapists are called on to do more and more, the ability to perform a complete history and physical exam may help the practitioner perform in alternative sites.

Once information has been gathered, the ability to share it with other health-care providers is essential for a seamless continuum of care. Documentation must be done in a way that facilitates the dissemination of information. Clear, concise, complete documentation is the key to multidisciplinary care of the patient.

Discussion Activities and Questions

1. How would you describe active listening?

2. How would you define adventitious breath sounds?

3. Auscultation can be performed when listening for breath sounds. Name another time in a full assessment when you would perform auscultation.

4. Define intimate space (using the definition from your textbook).

REVIEW

Multiple Choice

1. Bradycardia in adults is described as:

   a. >150 bpm
   b. <150 bpm and >112 bpm

   c. both a and b
   d. none of the above

2. Bradypnea in adults is:

   a. a respiratory rate below the normal range
   b. a respiratory rate above the normal range

   c. all of the above
   d. none of the above

3. Central cyanosis is present on a physical exam. In what part of the body is this present?

   a. the fingernail beds
   b. the lips

   c. the chest
   d. both b and c

4. Using a stethoscope to listen to sounds is called:

   a. percussion
   b. auscultation

   c. Glasgow coma test
   d. inspection

5. Gallop rhythm is an abnormal heart sound; it is so named because its sequence of sounds suggests the movement of what animal?

   a. rat
   b. horse

   c. frog
   d. none of the above

6. When performing a physical exam, you want to use close inspection with which of the senses?

   a. touch, sight, hearing, smell
   b. only taste
   c. only smell
   d. only sight
   e. b and c only
   f. all of the above

7. Kyphoscoliosis is associated with what body system?

   a. renal system
   b. GI system
   c. respiratory system
   d. skeletal system

8. Kyphosis is defined as:

   a. breathing pattern
   b. pulse pattern
   c. abnormal anteroposterior curvature
   d. both a and b

Lab Activities

1. Using small groups of four people, have each student introduce himself or herself to the others in the group, engaging the social space, personal space, and intimate space.

2. In the lab, pair up with a partner. Practice interviewing each other. Take about 10 minutes for each interview, and then report your findings. Tip: Use open-ended questions, such as "What brought you in here today?"

3. In lab groups of two, have students perform assessment skills, such as taking pulse, counting respiratory rate, taking blood pressure and pulse ox readings, and doing auscultation. Have each student report his or her findings. Tips:
   • Remember that this is the intimate space, so keep your voice steady and at a normal pitch.
   • Explain what you are doing every step of the way and brief your lab partner on your findings.
   • To help build trust, ask if your partner has any questions.

CHAPTER 14

Radiology for the Respiratory Therapist

INTRODUCTION

A respiratory therapist should be able to effectively review and analyze radiographic studies, should know how various imaging modalities can contribute to a patient's diagnosis and treatment, and should be able to use the information obtained from medical imaging to improve patient care. Such a knowledgeable RT is an asset to patients, to other health-care workers, and to the health-care facilities at which they work. To properly use medical imaging information, a respiratory therapist must understand the basic principles of how the study is created and how to systematically evaluate studies for their technical quality and meaning. Proficiency can be obtained and maintained only through frequent practice and learning from mentors and teachers.

Discussion Activities and Questions

1. A patient is admitted with acute congestive heart failure. What is likely to be seen on this patient's chest X-ray?

   On the patients chest X-ray, we would recognize a butterfly-shape.

2. List some differences between regular and portable X-rays. *Portable X-rays are done when patients are impossible to move; usually in the ER or ICU departments. although the portables are useful to get an idea of what is going on with the patient, the care-giver must be aware that the image was done on a portable X-ray because they do have limitations. Regular X-rays are always of better quality.*

217

3. List what could be detected on the X-ray of a patient with a suspected tension pneumothorax.

With a suspected tension pneumothorax, we could see a tracheal & mediastinal shift away from the affected side. and a mediastinal shift

4. List some reasons why it could be beneficial for a respiratory therapist to have a basic understanding of chest radiographs.

a resp. therapist could have the opportunity to evaluate the patient and treat any urgent issues prior to a physician being available.

Thought Questions

1. A 64-year-old patient presents to the Emergency Department in marked respiratory distress. The patient uses oxygen at home but has been getting progressively more short of breath. The patient is sitting in a tripod position and doing pursed-lip breathing. Discuss what types of findings might be seen on this patient's chest X-ray.

If the patient is in the tripod position & doing pursed-lip breathing, we know that they are in severe distress and we would most likely see a flat diaphram and widening of intercostal spaces in an X-ray.

2. A patient is exhibiting signs and symptoms of a possible pulmonary embolism. Discuss the best radiographic test to use to help confirm these suspicions. Would a chest X-ray be beneficial in this case?

a chest X-ray would not to beneficial, but a spiral CT would because it is an advanced X-ray that creates a data set w/ no gaps which makes it possible to see great detail in very small structures like the pulmonary and coronary arteries. This would allow a caregiver to recognize pulmonary emboli.

3. Is it beneficial to obtain alternative views in addition to the primary X-ray test that is ordered? If yes, explain why.

Yes, especially if we suspect a problem. An extra or alternative view could lead us to view something that may not have been in the first image. Expanding the view would always be beneficial.

REVIEW

Multiple Choice

1. A chest X-ray that displays tracheal and mediastinal shift toward one side is associated with:

   a. pneumonia
   b. asthma

   c. tension pneumothorax
   d. ARDS

2. What pattern could be detected on the chest X-ray of a patient with ARDS?

   a. ground-glass appearance
   b. butterfly pattern

   c. blunted costaphrenic angles
   d. hyperlucency

3. What is the best X-ray test to help detect pleural fluid in the lung?

   a. AP exam
   b. PA exam

   c. lateral neck
   d. lateral decubitus

4. What test could be used to determine narrowing or stenosis in blood vessels?

   a. ultrasound
   b. Doppler sonography

   c. needle biopsy
   d. 12-lead ECG

5. When evaluating for an aortic aneurysm, what would you look for on the X-ray?

   a. ground-glass appearance
   b. butterfly pattern

   c. tracheal shift
   d. dilation or ballooning appearance of aorta

6. A portable chest X-ray is:

   a. shot from back to front
   b. shot from front to back

   c. shot with the patient lying on one side
   d. rarely used

7. A flail chest is defined as?

   a. blood in the pleural space
   b. volume loss in the lung

   c. multiple fractures of adjacent ribs
   d. pleural fluid in the lung

Matching

Match these terms with their definitions on the right.

_C_ 1. lateral decubitus

_d_ 2. V/Q scan

_e_ 3. ultrasound

_b_ 4. atelectasis

_a_ 5. hemothorax

a. blood in pleural space

b. volume loss in lung

c. lying with affected side down

d. used to detect embolism

e. using sound waves to record images

Lab Activity

1. Students should review many different types of X-rays. Review the different types of respiratory diseases and what X-ray findings are commonly associated with them. In addition, students should familiarize themselves with how to look at an X-ray and what to look for. Present and discuss scenarios that discuss what X-ray view would be the most appropriate given the situation.

Clinical Laboratory Studies

INTRODUCTION

The respiratory therapist must have a basic understanding of chemistry and the various properties of atoms, bonds, and the atomic structure of biological molecules. This knowledge is necessary to understand how electrolytes influence and control metabolic reactions. Both sodium in the intracellular space and potassium in the extracellular space have a major influence on the distribution and retention of body fluids and on osmolality. Thus, electrolytes and body fluids affect changes in HCO_3^-, PCO_2, and pH.

Also helpful is an understanding of the various factors that control the concentration of both anions and cations in the body. Ionized calcium and ionized magnesium have been shown to be better indicators of cardiac function after cardiopulmonary bypass than the total levels of calcium and magnesium, consisting of both bound and free forms.

Respiratory therapists must be familiar with the various cardiac markers and their release into the blood.

The understanding of basic quality control, along with basic concepts of measuring various analytes, allows the respiratory therapist to monitor the accuracy of analytical results. Thus, proper and accurate information is provided to the physician or health-care provider.

Discussion Activities and Questions

1. Describe the three fluid compartments in the body. Intracellular fluid is water which is the most abundant compound in the body. Water is held in individual cellular compartments. Extracellular fluid is the water outside of the cells. Plasma is also a fluid compartment that is extracellular but has subcompartments that carry electrolytes.

2. What is meant by insensible water loss? How and where does it occur? Insensible water loss means that it is not able to be measured. This occurs substantially through perspiration, what we exhale and in feces. The average adult loses 1500-2000 mL daily.

3. You are seeing a patient who has an endotracheal tube in place. Explain how the presence of the tube can potentially affect fluid balance.

The endotracheal tube bypasses the upper airway where our natural humidification takes place, so a patient with a trach will have fluid loss. As a resp. therapist, we will be treating trach patients with humidity.

4. Explain the chloride shift.

When HCO_3 leaves the red blood cell, it must be replaced by another anion because the body makes constant effort to maintain electro-neutrality.

5. Explain why patients experiencing asthma attacks sometimes benefit from the administration of magnesium sulfate.

Pt's may experience muscle spasms in smooth airway muscle and this is sometimes caused by low magnesium levels.

6. Describe flame photometry and spectral analysis.

7. What is a biosensor?

PG. 218
for ?'s
for 7-11

8. Compare methods for measuring plasma chloride levels.

9. Explain why analytical instruments must be monitored for quality control.

10. What is the difference between standard deviation and coefficient of variance?

11. What is the value of trend analysis?

REVIEW

True or False

___T___   1. The lungs contribute to the body's insensible water loss.

___F___   2. Chloride is the most plentiful electrolyte in the body.

___T___   3. Cardiac arrest may be the consequence when potassium concentrations exceed 7.0 mmol/L.

___F___   4. Elevated chloride levels are associated with metabolic alkalosis.

___T___   5. Changes in bicarbonate levels will also change the plasma concentration of carbon dioxide.

___F___   6. Ionized calcium is calcium that is bound to proteins or diffusable ligands.

___T___   7. Plasma phosphorus levels are normally inversely related to the calcium levels.

___T___   8. Biosensors are devices that combine ion-specific electrodes, enzymatic methodology, and solid-phase technology to selectively recognize an element with a transducer.

___F___   9. When oxygen diffuses across the membrane of a Clark electrode, it is reduced at the anode.

___T___ 10. Precision is a measure of reproducibility.

___F___ 11. The scatter of control values should be evenly distributed above and below the mean.

Multiple Choice

1. The highest concentration of potassium in the body is in which of the following?

   a. plasma
   b. intracellular fluid
   c. red blood cells
   d. interstitial fluid

2. Intracellular water makes up what percent of total body weight?

   a. 20
   b. 30
   c. 40
   d. 60

3. The average daily insensible water loss for an adult is which of the following?

   a. 500–1000 mL
   b. 1000–1500 mL
   c. 1500–2000 mL
   d. 2000–2500 mL

4. The regulation of which of the following strongly influences the kidney's ability to retain water?

   a. Cl
   b. HCO_3
   c. K
   d. Na

5. Weakness, numbness, and cardiac abnormalities are most likely to occur with high plasma concentrations of which of the following?

   a. potassium
   b. sodium
   c. chloride
   d. calcium

6. A patient states that he is losing his sense of touch and has a decreased sensitivity to pain. This may be the result of which of the following?

   a. hyponatremia
   b. hypercalcemia
   c. hypermagnesemia
   d. hypokalemia

7. Which of the following is most likely to be a potential consequence of hypernatremia?

   a. respiratory acidosis
   b. edematous tissue
   c. decreased muscle contractility
   d. metabolic alkalosis

8. The PCO_2 electrode is basically which of the following?

   a. modified pH electrode
   b. permeable only to HCO_3
   c. permeable only to O_2
   d. an adapted lactate biosensor

9. Laboratory findings in compensated respiratory alkalosis include which of the following?

   a. decreased bicarbonate
   b. increased pH
   c. increased PO_2
   d. increased glucose

10. You are running control solutions on a blood gas analyzer. One of the controls comes in outside of acceptable limits. Which of the following is your best immediate course of action?

    a. take the analyzer out of service and call the service technician
    b. run a second control
    c. note the discrepancy and continue to run samples
    d. take recommended corrective action

Matching

Match the electrolyte with its normal range.

_e_ 1. Na

_c_ 2. Cl

_a_ 3. K

_b_ 4. HCO3

_d_ 5. Ca

a. 3.5–5.0

b. 22–26

c. 97–108

d. 8.5–10.0

e. 135–145

Lab Activities

1. Compare the blood gas analyzers at different hospitals in your area.

   a. What types do they have?

   b. Who does the analysis (i.e., is respiratory care or the lab responsible)?

   c. What quality control procedures do they have in place?

2. Look at the following graph.

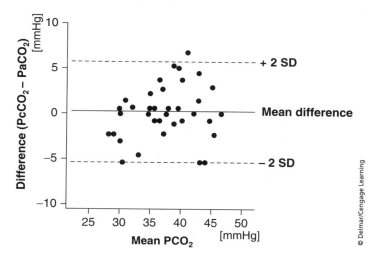

a. What is it?

b. What is it used for?

Arterial Blood Gases and Noninvasive Monitoring of Oxygen and Carbon Dioxide

INTRODUCTION

Arterial blood gas values are a key diagnostic tool in many diseases and conditions. They allow the measurement and analysis of acid–base balance. This technique involves the examination and determination of pH, $PaCO_2$, and HCO_3^-. By examining the ratios of acid ($PaCO_2$) and base (HCO_3^-) in relation to the pH, respiratory therapists can, at least broadly, determine the source of acid–base disturbances. With knowledge of the anion gap, they can further define these alterations in acid–base homeostasis. Acid-base and blood gas physiology are among respiratory care's most important knowledge bases. Many times the respiratory therapists are the experts in this area, and their knowledge is critical for the survival of the patient.

ABGs can be measured directly by invasive sampling and direct analysis of blood and noninvasively and indirectly through the use of sophisticated devices such as photospectrometers and pulse oximeters. Some of the methods and devices used, such as blood gas analyzers, provide actual measured data; others, such as the capnograph, provide data that are more valuable when looking at trends over time. Remember that ABGs are like a static picture, giving a look at the respiratory physiology at a single second in time. Trend data are more like a video, enabling the RT to see how the physiology has acted over time. So the choice becomes the desirability of a static glimpse at the ABG values or a dynamic presentation of real-time physiology under current conditions.

Arterial blood gas procurement, analysis, and interpretation are skills that must be learned, practiced, and evaluated repeatedly over time. In addition to maintaining current skill levels, the respiratory therapist must be aware that blood gas analysis technology, techniques, and procedures are constantly being upgraded and improved. Such change only further emphasizes the need for continuous training in this area of respiratory therapist practice. An ongoing program of quality assurance, remediation, and review is a mandatory part of offering a blood gas service.

Discussion Activities and Questions

1. List the steps in the TCA cycle.

2. According to the Henderson-Hasselbalch equation, pH = _____ .

3. List the four basic methods of buffering H^+ in the body.

4. Describe the Allen's test.

5. Discuss the shortcomings of pulse oximetry.

6. Discuss the origin of normal lab values. Are they perhaps biased toward a particular population?

7. What is plethysmography?

8. A patient who has just been rescued from a very smoky fire is transported to the ED. He is in mild respiratory distress and his lips and skin appear almost cherry red. Carbon monoxide exposure is suspected. However, his SpO_2 on room air is 100%. How do you account for this?

9. Explain the difference between mainstream and sidestream capnography.

10. Draw and label a normal capnogram.

11. Explain why transcutaneous PaO_2 monitoring is generally more effective on neonates than on adults.

12. Describe the hemoglobin molecule.

13. Explain the significance of the anion gap.

14. Describe at least two emerging technologies related to the monitoring of ventilation and/or oxygenation.

REVIEW

True or False

—— 1. Respiration refers to the gross movement of gas into and out of the lungs.

—— 2. Hyperventilation is defined as a respiratory rate greater than 30 breaths per minute.

—— 3. Capillary sampling is not arterial blood sampling.

—— 4. SpO_2 is a poor indicator of ventilation status.

—— 5. TcO_2 and $TcCO_2$ always correlate with PaO_2 and $PaCO_2$.

—— 6. Looking at a capnogram can aid in the detection of bronchospasm.

—— 7. Capnography is not a strong predictor of postresuscitation survival.

—— 8. Overuse of antacids can shift the pH into the acidotic range.

—— 9. The Severinghaus electrode is a miniaturized polarographic electrode.

—— 10. The Sanz electrode assesses the concentration of H^+.

—— 11. The pulse oximeter is the best tool to use to monitor oxygenation during a cardiac arrest.

—— 12. Normal hemoglobin levels for adult males are 12.0–16.0 g/dL.

—— 13. Icing a blood sample that will be used for electrolyte analysis will yield inaccurate results for some of the electrolytes.

Multiple Choice

1. The byproduct of aerobic metabolism is which of the following?

   a. carbon dioxide
   b. glucose

   c. lactic acid
   d. hydrogen ions

2. Hyperventilation is the body's initial response to which of the following?

   a. respiratory alkalosis
   b. respiratory acidosis

   c. metabolic alkalosis
   d. metabolic acidosis

3. Acidemia is defined as a pH:

   a. less than 7.35
   b. greater than 7.45

   c. less than 7.20
   d. greater than 7.50

4. Just prior to performing an arterial puncture on a 60-year-old patient, you perform the Allen's test on the left wrist. The result of the test is negative. Based on this, which of the following should be your next step?

   a. Perform the puncture.
   b. Evaluate the right radial.

   c. Notify the physician.
   d. Perform the puncture on the left brachial.

5. You are attempting an arterial puncture on a 42-year-old patient via the right radial. You feel a good pulse; however, during repositioning, you inadvertently withdraw the needle completely from the skin. Which of the following is your best course of action?

   a. Immediately reinsert the needle.
   b. Attempt the puncture on a different artery.

   c. Change needles and reinsert.
   d. Quit and notify your supervisor.

6. You are preparing to obtain blood from an arterial line that is in the patient's left radial artery. Which of the following do you need in addition to the standard equipment you would use for an arterial puncture?

   a. extra syringe
   b. capillary tubes

   c. Betadine swabs
   d. heparin

7. A HCO_3^- of 34 mmol/dL would be classified as which of the following?

   a. normal
   b. respiratory alkalosis

   c. metabolic alkalosis
   d. metabolic acidosis

8. A patient who has had a very recent hip replacement self-administers a large dose of morphine to ease the pain (via patient-controlled analgesia PCA pump). This could possibly induce which of the following?

   a. respiratory acidosis
   b. respiratory alkalosis

   c. metabolic acidosis
   d. metabolic alkalosis

9. A patient presents to the Emergency Department after having consumed an unknown quantity of anti-freeze. He has the following blood gas data:

pH	7.20
$PaCO_2$	29
HCO_3^-	12
PaO_2	220 (on 50% oxygen)

   Which of the following is the best treatment for this patient?

   a. increase the oxygen
   b. mechanical ventilation

   c. sodium bicarbonate
   d. respiratory stimulants

10. A patient has just undergone major abdominal surgery. Currently, she is in the ICU. She is receiving mechanical ventilation and has a nasogastric tube in place attached to suction. She has the following blood gas data:

pH	7.58
$PaCO_2$	30
HCO_3^-	29
PaO_2	96 (on 40% oxygen)

    Which of the following is the best interpretation of her acid–base state?

    a. normal
    b. respiratory alkalosis

    c. metabolic acidosis
    d. mixed alkalosis

11. The best way to correct the acid–base problem in question 10 is which of the following?

    a. Administer sodium bicarbonate.
    b. Decrease the ventilator minute volume.

    c. Stop the gastric suction.
    d. No correction is necessary.

12. A patient who has been hemorrhaging from a severe leg wound is transported to the ED. He has a thready pulse. The SpO_2 (taken via finger sensor) is 75%. The patient is receiving 100% oxygen and is in no respiratory distress. Which of the following is the best explanation for the low SpO_2?

   a. motion artifact

   b. light interference

   c. low perfusion

   d. the patient is extremely hypoxemic

Lab Activities

1. Using a calculator with a log function, calculate the pH if the $PaCO_2$ is 52 mm Hg and the HCO_3^- is 18 mmol/dL.

2. On a partner, find the following arteries (pulses):

   a. radial

   b. brachial

   c. dorsalis pedis

3. Once you have found the radial artery on your partner, perform the Allen's test.

4. At home, find your own femoral artery (pulse).

5. Practice arterial puncture on an appropriate training device (e.g., dedicated arterial puncture arm). If possible, practice using both your dominant and nondominant hands.

6. Measure the SpO_2 and pulse on a partner using both the fingers and the toes.

7. Try measuring the SpO_2 on the same partner after he or she has put nail polish on one of the fingers. Try different shades (e.g., red, black, white, etc.). What did you observe?

8. With your instructor, survey the various hospitals in your area for the following:

   a. Do they use transcutaneous monitoring? If so, why do they use it?

   b. Do they routinely use capnometry and/or capnography? If so, how do they use it?

   c. Do they use point-of-care testing? If so, which analyzers do they use and what do they measure?

CHAPTER 17

Pulmonary Function Testing

INTRODUCTION

In pulmonary function testing, spirometry or the forced vital capacity measurements are used to find out whether the subject's lung function is normal or abnormal. Abnormal findings indicate a need for further testing to assess the type and degree of lung impairment. Such tests include lung volumes, diffusing capacity, postbronchodilator spirometry, maximum voluntary ventilation, airway resistance, lung compliance, the nitrogen washout gas distribution test, and the CO_2 response curve. Specialized test regimens, such as cardiopulmonary stress testing and broncho-provocation, help assess the severity of lung disorders.

Equipment should be calibrated on a regular basis according to manufacturers' recommendations. Spirometers should have quality assurance assessments quarterly to ensure their accuracy. Infection control is easy to achieve by the use of disposable mouthpieces and noseclips and the sterilization of nondisposable items after each use. Handwashing is, of course, important after handling equipment and between subjects.

Discussion Activities and Questions

1. List two reasons for performing pulmonary function testing.

2. Describe the major components of pulmonary function testing.

3. List four examples of a restrictive disease.

4. Draw and label a normal flow-volume loop.

5. Draw and label a flow-volume loop for a person with severe airway obstruction.

6. Briefly describe the three methods of measuring FRC. Which is the least accurate? Why?

7. During the helium dilution test for measuring FRC, the patient begins to get progressively more short of breath, seeming to breathe faster and deeper. What might cause this reaction?

8. Discuss why carbon monoxide is used in the test for diffusing capacity. Why is this not dangerous?

9. What is meant by "anaerobic threshold"?

10. Describe the procedure for a cardiopulmonary stress test.

11. What is the purpose of a bronchoprovocation test?

12. List three types of spirometers. Which is the most commonly used?

REVIEW

True or False

_____ 1. A patient recently diagnosed with amyotrophic lateral sclerosis should have a pulmonary function test performed.

_____ 2. The condition of the airways is assessed using volumes.

_____ 3. Functional residual capacity can be measured via spirometry.

_____ 4. To obtain good results when pulmonary function tests are performed, the patient must be fully cooperative.

_____ 5. Dentures should be removed prior to performing any pulmonary function test.

_____ 6. When determining the validity of PFT results, the ATS (American Thoracic Society) recommends at least two acceptable maneuvers be saved.

_____ 7. If a patient is receiving Advair, it should be stopped at least 24 hours prior to pulmonary function testing.

_____ 8. The gas mixture used when measuring diffusing capacity contains 3% CO.

_____ 9. Diffusing capacity will often be decreased in pulmonary fibrosis.

_____ 10. Lung compliance can be measured using body plethysmography.

Multiple Choice

1. When determining predicted values for patients undergoing pulmonary function testing, the equations generally require which of the following?

      1. body mass index
      2. height
      3. age
      4. sex

  a. 1, 2
  b. 1, 4
                    c. 2, 3, 4
                    d. 3

2. Given the following data, calculate the TLC.

    V_T 600 mL
    FRC   2400 mL
    IRV   2000 mL

  a. 3.0 L
  b. 4.4 L
                    c. 5.0 L
                    d. 5.6 L

3. Which of the following can be measured via spirometry?

  a. FRC
  b. RV
                    c. TLC
                    d. VC

4. Which of the following is a critical element in obtaining good results when performing spirometry?

  a. coaching
  b. patient's ability to stand
                    c. clean, quiet environment
                    d. patient's ability to read

5. Look at the flow-volume loop in the following figure. Which of the following is the best interpretation?

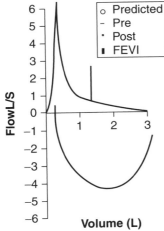

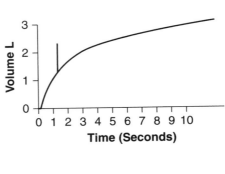

© Delmar/Cengage Learning

a. obstructive

b. restrictive

c. mixed obstructive and restrictive

d. normal

6. You are working the night shift at the hospital. One of your patients is scheduled for a pulmonary function test at 0900. The patient receives albuterol via small volume nebulizer q 4 hours. So as not to interfere with the test, which of the following is the latest time the patient should receive his aerosol treatment?

a. 0400

b. 0500

c. 0600

d. 0700

7. A patient performs an FEV_1 maneuver before and after administration of a bronchodilator. Based on the data below, what is the percent improvement?

Pre-bronchodilator

Actual	*Predicted*	*% Predicted*
2.8 L	4.4 L	64%

Post-bronchodilator

Actual	Predicted	% Predicted
3.6	4.4	82%

a. 10%

b. 14%

c. 18%

d. 29%

8. Which of the following is the best interpretation for the spirometry data below?

Parameter	*% Predicted*
FVC	79%
FEV_1	42%
$FEV_{1\%}$	50%
$FEF_{25-75\%}$	12%

a. normal

b. mixed obstructrive and restrictive

c. obstructive

d. restrictive

9. In measuring FRC, the test usually begins at what point?

a. end of a normal exhalation

b. end of a maximal exhalation

c. end of a normal inhalation

d. beginning of a tidal breath

10. Prior to performing a bronchoprovocation test, anticholinergic drugs should be withheld for a minimum of how long?

a. 4 hours

b. 6 hours

c. 8 hours

d. 12 hours

Lab Activities

1. Survey the hospitals in your area.

    a. Who does bedside spirometry?

    b. Who does complete pulmonary function testing?

2. Practice performing spirometry on multiple partners. Test with and without coaching. Did you notice a difference in any of the values? Why?

3. Compare the peak flow obtained via spirometry with the peak flow obtained via peak flowmeter.

4. Interpret the following data:

Date:
Name:

Pulmonary Function Lab

ID:

Gender	Height(cm):	Weight(kg):	Age	Room: Body Mass Index			
Medication Physician		Technician		Smoker Quit		How Long Stopped:	yrs

			#7 Ref	#8 CI	#9 Pre	#10 % Ref	#11 Post	#12 % Ref	#13 %Chg
Spirometry									
#1	FVC	Liters	3.19	(2.5 − 3.9)	(2.33)	(73)	(2.30)	(72)	−1
#2	FEV1	Liters	2.62	(2.1 − 3.2)	(1.01)	(39)	(1.01)	(38)	−0
#3	FEV1/FVC	%	82	(72.8 − 90.7)	(43)		(44)		
	FEV1/SVC	%			40				
	FEF25-75%	L/sec	2.85	(1.5 − 4.2)	(0.40)	(14)	(0.38)	(13)	−6
	FEF50%	L/sec	3.50	(1.7 − 5.3)	(0.46)	(13)	(0.39)	(11)	−16
	PEF	L/sec	5.85	(3.0 − 8.7)	3.88	68	3 − 88	63	−5
	FET100%	Sec			9.61		11.08		15
	FIF50%	L/sec	5.50		2.14	39	2.68	49	26
	FEF/FIF50				0.22		0.14		−33
	FVL ECode				000010		000010		
Lung Volumes									
#4	TLC	Liters	4.90	(3.8 − 6.0)	(5.99)	(122)			
	VC	Liters	3.19	(2.5 − 3.9)	2.55	80			
	IC	Liters	2.10	(1.7 − 2.5)	1.87	89			
	FRC PL	Liters	2.73	(1.7 − 3.8)	(4.12)	(151)			
	ERV	Liters	1.00		0.62	62			
#5	RV	Liters	1.74	(1.0 − 2.5)	(3.43)	(198)			
	RV/TLC	%	35	(24.2 − 46.2)	(57)				
	LVol ECode				000002				
Diffusing Capacity									
#6	DLCO	mL/mmHg/min	22.3	(15.8 − 28.8)	16.4	74			
	DL Adj	mL/mmHg/min	22.3	(15.8 − 28.8)	16.4	74			
	DLCO/VA	mL/mmHg/min/L	5.33	4.0 − 6.6	(3.75)	(70)			
	DLCO ECode			(3.8 − 6.0)	0000				
	TLC Sb	Liters	4.90		4.37	89			

Comments: #14

TESTS ARE PRE AND POST SALBUTAMOL 4 PUFFS

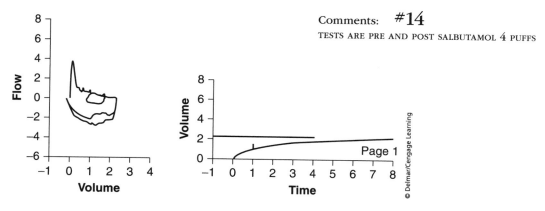

Page 1

© Delmar/Cengage Learning

CHAPTER 18

Polysomnography and Other Tests for Sleep Disorders

INTRODUCTION

Normal sleep consists of alternating periods of rapid eye movement and nonrapid eye movement sleep. Sleep patterns and stages can be observed by using EEG, EOG, and EMG and by monitoring breathing and arterial oxygen saturation. The resulting data can be interpreted to detect the presence of sleep disorders, including sleep-disordered breathing, narcolepsy, and periodic limb movements in sleep.

The polysomnogram is used to report sleep data. The therapist sets filters and sensitivities for the equipment used and prepares the patient for the testing, including patient or biological calibration to ensure accurate data collection and minimal artifact. The therapist also monitors the test in progress. The data collected are scored or interpreted to determine whether any sleep disorders are present.

Effective forms of therapy for sleep-disordered breathing include continuous positive airway pressure, in which positive pressure established in the patient's airway acts as a pneumatic splint to keep the airway open. CPAP may be applied with a mask or other device, depending on the patient's needs and tolerance. The amount of pressure must be titrated to produce maximum therapeutic results while maintaining patient comfort. Bilevel positive airway pressure allows inspiratory and expiratory pressure levels to be adjusted independently, and autotitrating CPAP devices automatically adjust pressure according to patient requirements.

Discussion Activities and Questions

1. What is the difference between CPAP and bilevel PAP therapy?

2. What is the normal pattern of sleep architecture throughout the night?

3. What are some respiratory and cardiovascular changes that happen during sleep?

Thought Question

1. A patient having a sleep study shows signs of having obstructive sleep apnea. A second study is ordered using CPAP titration. The patient states that she is extremely claustrophobic and has no interest in wearing any type of mask. What steps can you take to help reassure the patient and to convince her to try CPAP?

REVIEW

Multiple Choice

1. The sleep disorder most commonly encountered in the sleep lab is:

   a. central sleep apnea
   b. obstructive sleep apnea
   c. narcolepsy
   d. sleep deprivation

2. What are some common side effects related to use of CPAP?

   a. difficulty exhaling
   b. nasal dryness
   c. nasal congestion
   d. a and b
   e. all of the above

3. The test most commonly used to assess sleepiness is:

   a. multiple sleep latency
   b. autotitration
   c. bilevel therapy
   d. polysomnography

4. Slow wave or delta sleep is associated with:

   a. N1 stage
   b. N2 stage
   c. N3 stage
   d. NREM stage

5. A graphical representation of the sleep stages is called a:

   a. polygraph
   b. EMG
   c. EOG
   d. sleep histogram

6. Sleep disturbed by frequent arousals is called:

   a. deprivation
   b. fragmentation
   c. latency
   d. architecture

7. Which of the following statements concerning periodic limb movements in sleep is true?

   a. occurs during the latter half of the night
   b. commonly found in REM sleep
   c. a person can have PLMS even if he or she does not have RLS symptoms
   d. frequency increases in the elderly population

8. If there is a paradoxical pattern between the chest and abdominal signals, it should be scored as a/an:

   a. obstructive apnea
   b. mixed apnea

   c. central apnea
   d. mixed hypopnea

Matching

Match these terms with their definitions on the right.

_____ 1. apnea

_____ 2. cataplexy

_____ 3. epoch

_____ 4. artifact

_____ 5. hypnogogic

a. sudden loss of muscle tone

b. activity that interferes with the signal

c. absence of airflow for at least 10 seconds

d. hallucinations upon awakening

e. 30-second sleep periods

Lab Activity

1. In the lab, students should be familiarized with many of the different types of CPAP and bilevel PAP devices that are available, and shown how to adjust the pressures on these machines. In addition, a variety of CPAP masks, ranging from pillows to nasal and full-face masks should be displayed with the opportunity for the students to fit each other with different styles of masks to determine which one would be more suitable. This will be invaluable, as they will face many situations during their careers in which they must try to find a mask acceptable to a patient. In addition, they will encounter numerous styles of machines and masks; the lab is a good place for students to familiarize themselves with some of the types and styles they may use later on.

CHAPTER 19

Cardiac and Hemodynamic Monitoring

INTRODUCTION

Managing the critically ill patient in the clinical setting requires a complete assessment of the patient's cardiac status. Noninvasive assessment includes determining the patient's heart rate and rhythm and correlating them with the presence and quality of peripheral pulses. In addition, a quick check of the patient's capillary refill, skin color and temperature, level of consciousness, urine output, and neck veins determines whether further invasive monitoring is necessary. With the use of invasive catheters, important hemodynamic parameters can be measured directly: oxygenation, cardiac output, central venous pressure, pulmonary artery pressure, pulmonary capillary wedge pressure, and arterial pressure. With the information obtained from the invasive catheters, additional parameters can be calculated (mean pressures, vascular resistance, and ventricular stroke work index), allowing for the optimal use of medications to maintain hemodynamic stability.

Discussion Activities and Questions

1. What is the importance of monitoring mixed venous oxygenation?

2. List some noninvasive methods of assessing a patient's hemodynamic status.

3. Identify the lethal rhythm shown in the following figure:

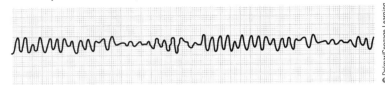

4. What is the heart rate of the rhythm shown in the following figure? Assume that this is a 6-second strip.

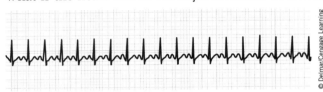

REVIEW

Multiple Choice

1. AV block with a normal QRS duration is associated with:

   a. complete heart block
   b. type I AV block

   c. Mobitz type II AV block
   d. 2:1 AV block

2. Which category of premature ventricular contractions is considered less serious?

   a. multifocal PVCs
   b. couplets of PVCs

   c. three or more PVCs in a row
   d. R on T PVCs

3. Which factor listed has an effect on cardiac afterload?

   a. venous return
   b. duration of diastole
   c. atrial contraction
   d. blood volume and viscosity

4. The primary pacemaker of the heart is the:

   a. AV node
   b. bundle of His
   c. Purkinje fiber
   d. SA node

5. The standard color of electrode for the left arm on an ECG machine is:

   a. green
   b. black
   c. white
   d. red

6. The period of contraction in a cardiac cycle is called:

   a. systole
   b. preload
   c. diastasis
   d. diastole

7. Cor pulmonale and Tetralogy of Fallot are diseases that may display which rhythm?

   a. premature ventricular contraction
   b. sinus bradycardia
   c. atrial flutter
   d. nonparoxysmal junctional tachycardia

8. Normal S_vO_2 is:

   a. 95–100%
   b. 12–15 mg
   c. 4–8 Lpm
   d. 60–80%

Matching

Match these terms with their definitions on the right.

—— 1. cardiac cycle

—— 2. afterload

—— 3. sinus bradycardia

—— 4. diastasis

—— 5. repolarization

a. SA node discharge <60 bpm

b. change in transmembrane potential from positive to negative

c. one complete heartbeat

d. force that ventricles work against to pump blood

e. ventricles slow to a standstill

Lab Activity

1. Possible lab activities for this chapter include practicing ECG electrode placement on either a mannequin or a male volunteer. Also, students could be shown various sample ECG strips and asked to identify the rhythm and calculate the rate, using the methods discussed in the chapter. A sample pulmonary artery catheter can be displayed along with a diagram of how the pulmonary artery catheter is placed.

Case Study

1. Mrs. Jones presents to the Emergency Room complaining of dizziness and fainting spells. After a quick assessment, an ECG is performed that yields the tracing in the following figure:

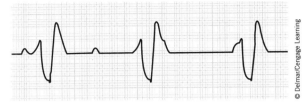

   a. What is this dysrhythmia?

   b. What is the relationship between the atria and the ventricles?

   c. Should this dysrhythmia be treated?

Essential Therapeutics

Oxygen and Medical Gas Therapy

INTRODUCTION

Medical gas therapy is an integral part of respiratory care practice. The competent, skilled practitioner is well versed in all aspects of therapy. Patient assessment and critical thinking skills are vital, as are skills in equipment selection and troubleshooting. The goals, indications, physiological effects, hazards, and side effects of therapy must always be considered and recognized. These factors, along with documented outcomes assessment, reflect not only a competent practitioner but also a professional one who is able to interact successfully with other members of the health-care team and to contribute actively to the diagnosis, treatment, and recovery of the patient.

Discussion Activities and Questions

1. Compare the density of oxygen with the density of helium. On the basis of this comparison, what is the advantage to a person with COPD in breathing a mixture of oxygen and helium?

2. Explain what happens if compressed gas cylinders are kept in very hot or very cold environments.

3. What are some characteristics and advantages of liquid versus gas bulk storage systems?

4. Compare the three safety systems for cylinder connecting devices.

5. Explain how a reducing valve works.

6. List at least five assessment parameters indicative of hypoxemia.

7. Describe the difference between low-flow and high-flow oxygen delivery devices.

8. When and how would you use a nonrebreathing mask?

9. List some primary purposes of hyperbaric medicine.

10. Explain how nitric oxide is used and the kinds of conditions for which it may be useful.

REVIEW

True or False

_____   1. The color of oxygen is green.

_____   2. The DOT requires hydrostatic testing of cylinders every 5 or 10 years.

_____   3. Fractional distillation is the most common and cost-effective method of producing oxygen.

_____   4. The only accurate way to measure liquid contents is to note the gauge pressure.

_____   5. The standard flowmeter used in oxygen outlets is a Bourdon tube.

_____   6. Infants are at risk for developing retinopathy of prematurity until one month of age.

_____   7. A patient receiving oxygen via a 28% air entrainment mask has a minute volume of 6 Lpm. The oxygen flowmeter is set at 8 Lpm. The total flow from the mask is sufficient for the patient.

_____   8. The FiO_2 produced by a nasal cannula running at a specific liter flow is fixed.

_____   9. If you want a patient to retain CO_2, the best device to use is a partial rebreathing mask.

_____ 10. Hyperbaric chambers increase the FiO_2 of the gas a patient breathes while in the chamber.

_____ 11. Arterial blood gas analysis is generally more accurate than pulse oximetry.

Multiple Choice

1. Which of the following is responsible for technical standards for manufacture terminology and testing procedures?

   a. ISO   c. OSHA
   b. DOT   d. FDA

2. You need to transport a patient to CT. The patient will require oxygen for the transport. What size oxygen cylinder are you most likely to use?

   a. A
   b. E
   c. H
   d. K

3. A cylinder that has a plus sign is normally filled to which of the following (in psi)?

   a. 1600
   b. 2000
   c. 2200
   d. 2500

4. Oxygen gas occupies a volume that is how many times that of liquid oxygen per cubic feet?

   a. 500
   b. 624
   c. 713
   d. 861

5. A person travels to the top of Pikes Peak and becomes hypoxemic. Which of the following is the most likely cause of the hypoxemia?

   a. diffusion defect
   b. low alveolar PO_2
   c. ventilation/perfusion mismatch
   d. shunt

6. To minimize the risk of oxygen toxicity, the FiO_2 should be kept below what level, if possible?

   a. .70
   b. .50
   c. .40
   d. .35

7. The transtracheal oxygen catheter requires approximately how much less oxygen than a nasal cannula?

   a. 10%
   b. 20%
   c. 30%
   d. 50%

8. All of the following are conditions for which hyperbaric medicine is potentially useful except:

   a. rheumatoid arthritis
   b. gas gangrene infection
   c. carbon monoxide poisoning
   d. thermal burns

9. A patient on helium–oxygen mixture of 80:20 requires a flow of 15 Lpm. The flowmeter should be set on which of the following?

   a. 6.5
   b. 8.3
   c. 10.4
   d. 15

Lab Activities

1. Consider your hospital experience.

   a. What flowmeters have you seen in the rooms?

   b. Is there a difference between the flowmeters used in medical-surgical rooms, the ED, and the ICU?

   c. Why?

2. Consider oxygen distribution and use in the hospitals you have visited.

   a. How is oxygen monitored in the hospital?

   b. What do you do in case of fire?

3. Describe the function and purpose of large-volume jet nebulizers. What are some ways you can increase the total flow of gas from such a device?

4. Discuss the uses and relative advantages of arterial blood gas analysis, pulse oximetry, and transcutaneous monitoring. Which do you see most often in the acute care hospital?

5. In 2008, a pulse oximeter with expanded measurement capability was introduced.

   a. What are some of these expanded measurement capabilities?

   b. What are the potential clinical applications?

6. Using some hospital-based oxygen protocols that you may have seen as a guide, construct your own basic protocol.

CHAPTER 21

Humidity and Aerosol Therapy

INTRODUCTION

Humidity is described in terms of its presence in our environment as absolute humidity (AH) and relative humidity (RH), according to the amount of water vapor present and expressed as water vapor content or water vapor pressure. Temperature affects a gas's ability to carry moisture: As temperature increases, a gas can carry more water vapor; as a gas cools, its capacity to carry water vapor decreases and condensation, or rainout, occurs.

This relation also pertains to inspired gas as it travels through the respiratory system. Humidity in the respiratory system, *body humidity*, is the water vapor content required to fully saturate alveolar air at normal body temperature. The difference between the body humidity and the absolute humidity of inspired air is called the *humidity deficit*.

Maintaining adequate humidity in the respiratory system is the role of the respiratory mucosal lining. When inspired gases are underhumidified, such as those that occur in the delivery of anhydrous gases, the mucosal lining must give up water to the inspired gas to reach body temperature pressure saturated (BTPS). Over time, this humidity deficit can lead to the retention of thick dried secretions, atelectasis, pneumonia, and pulmonary compromise. When inspired gas is overhumidified, as may occur when the gas contains aerosols or is at a temperature higher than body temperature, water drops out of suspension onto the mucosal lining, and excess body fluid is retained. This fluid retention leads to an increased depth of the aqueous sol layer and affects ciliary action in the removal of secretions.

Aerosols are liquid or solid particles that are suspended in a gas or a substance that contains such particles. Aerosols can occur naturally in the environment or in a chemical reaction, or they can be created artificially. How long an aerosol particle can remain in suspension depends on its size. Size, in turn, is affected by the temperature and RH of the carrier gas and by the tonicity of the solution being aerosolized. Equipment design determines the mass median aerodynamic diameter (MMAD) of the artificially created aerosol, thus determining its initial size. Aerosol stability is also influenced by the kinetic activity of the aerosol particle and the concentration of the particles. The instability of an aerosol particle in the respiratory tract leads to deposition in the upper or lower airway or in the lung parenchyma. Where deposition occurs and the type of agents being used determine the therapeutic effectiveness of the aerosolized solution.

The use of humidity devices in the clinical setting is the responsibility of the respiratory therapist and must be considered when administering dry medical gases. Supplemental humidity in low-flow systems that deliver gas to the upper airway should provide a minimum output of 10 mg/L, whereas a high-flow system delivering gas that bypasses the upper airway should provide a minimum of 30 mg/L. Hazards of humidity therapy include excessive delivery of heat and moisture, electrical malfunctions, and risk of infection. The effectiveness of humidity devices depends on the temperature of the water and gas, the length of contact time, and the surface area of the liquid-to-gas interface.

The types of low-flow humidity devices are various bubble humidifiers such as the diffuser and jet humidifier. High-flow devices are the passover and wick humidifiers and the heat and moisture exchangers. These systems can deliver humidity that is cool or heated using heating elements that are servocontrolled or nonservocontrolled. Systems such as the

Vapotherm and Aquinox are high-flow, high-humidity, heated systems designed for use with a nasal cannula. Heated wire circuits are an adjunct to humidification systems that attempt to eliminate the excess condensation due to changes in temperature within the ventilator circuit.

The use of aerosol-generating devices in the clinical setting requires a physician's order in most hospitals or a respiratory care department protocol to allow the respiratory therapist to choose the type of nebulizer that will meet the patient's needs. Aerosols are delivered as bland solutions or as medicated solutions, for intermittent therapy or continuous therapy, to achieve a variety of desired effects. Hazards of aerosol therapy are contamination, overhydration, swelling of dried secretions, medication side effects, and shock from electrically powered devices. Aerosol deposition in the airway is determined by the patient's ventilatory pattern, the integrity of the airway, nebulizer design, and delivery device. The types of aerosol generators are bulb nebulizers, dry powder inhalers, metered-dose inhalers, small-volume nebulizers, large-volume nebulizers, ultrasonic nebulizers, Babbington nebulizers, and small-particle aerosol generator (SPAG) units.

The respiratory therapist must understand the principles of hydration of the respiratory tract to maintain a humidity balance in a patient's airways and must determine the need for medication delivery to the airways of the compromised patient. In aerosol and humidity therapy, selecting the most appropriate device, monitoring the functioning of the device, assessing the patient, and making any necessary changes are the responsibilities of the respiratory therapist.

Discussion Activities and Questions

1. Explain the concept of relative humidity.

2. What is body humidity?

3. What is the definition of "aerosol"?

4. What happens to aerosol particles that are introduced into a gas stream that is warmer and more humid?

5. What is meant by "bland aerosol"?

6. What precautions should be taken when attaching a patient to a humidification device?

7. What is the advantage of using a heated wire circuit?

8. Describe the four basic designs of heat and moisture exchangers.

9. Compare the use of and specifications for two different types of high-flow nasal cannulas.

10. Describe the ideal breathing pattern for a patient to use during aerosol therapy via small-volume nebulizer.

REVIEW

True or False

—— 1. Water vapor content is often expressed as mg/L.

—— 2. Cooler air holds less water vapor than warmer air.

—— 3. Mucus is 85% water.

—— 4. At BTPS, condensation occurs in the inspired gas.

—— 5. Smog is a type of aerosol.

—— 6. Nebulized hypertonic saline is an example of a bland aerosol.

—— 7. The physician will nearly always order humidification of nasal oxygen.

—— 8. It is not necessary to remove the HME from the ventilator circuit during aerosol therapy.

—— 9. Cool aerosols tend to cause more airway reactivity than heated aerosols.

—— 10. Small-volume nebulizers cannot be used with neonates.

Multiple Choice

1. Which of the following is used to measure relative humidity?

   a. hygrometer
   b. barometer
   c. anometer
   d. galvanometer

2. Which of the following is a hallmark sign of overhydration?

   a. decreased breath sounds
   b. thin, watery secretions
   c. scattered crackles
   d. systemic hypertension

3. You want to administer an aerosol that will absorb water from the surrounding tissues. Which of the following would be best to use?

   a. 3% saline
   b. isotonic saline
   c. pure water
   d. 0.45% saline

4. You need to deliver a drug that will penetrate to the alveolar level. What is the largest particle size that will accomplish this (in μm)?

   a. 0.5
   b. 3
   c. 5
   d. 7

5. You receive an order to administer 3% saline to a patient in order to induce sputum. Which of the following devices would be best to use?

   a. small particle aerosol generator
   b. large-volume nebulizer
   c. Babbington
   d. ultrasonic

6. A patient has been receiving oxygen via nasal cannula at 4 Lpm for about 24 hours. She is complaining of a dry nose and throat. Which of the following is your best course of action?

   a. Add a bubble humidifier.
   b. Recommend that she increase her fluid intake.
   c. Change the cannula to a 35% air entrainment mask.
   d. Change the cannula to an aerosol mask connected to a 40% LVN.

7. Which of the following is the best possible indication for a bland, cool aerosol?

   a. thick tenacious secretions
   b. upper airway swelling
   c. bronchoconstriction
   d. pneumonia

8. Which of the following is a relative disadvantage of dry powder inhalers?

   a. They are only available with inhaled corticosteroids.
   b. The patient must generate a high inspiratory flow rate.
   c. They are best used with a valved holding chamber.
   d. They must be cleaned with soapy water after each use.

9. Which of the following are steps a patient should follow when using a metered dose inhaler?

   1. Shake the canister prior to actuation.
   2. Breathe in fast after actuation.
   3. Hold breath for several seconds following actuation.
   4. Take the second puff immediately after the first.

   a. 1, 2, 4
   b. 1, 3
   c. 2, 3, 4
   d. 3, 4

10. You receive an order to administer continuous albuterol to a patient who is having a severe asthma attack. Which of the following would be best to use?

    a. HEART nebulizer
    b. USN
    c. LVN
    d. SVN

Lab Activities

1. Review the factors that make up the mucociliary system:

   a. What are the components of the system?

   b. What is the composition of mucus?

c. What are some disorders that can interfere with normal mucociliary function?

2. You need to administer a bronchodilator to a patient who is experiencing an asthma attack. Explain the factors you will need to consider in administering the medication, including the MMAD.

3. Consider the respiratory therapy departments you have seen in your experience. Assuming that these departments were responsible for administering aerosolized drugs:

   a. What kinds of devices did they have for this purpose?

   b. What are the specifications of these devices (e.g., MMAD, etc.)?

   c. Do you believe that the devices were of a type that could deliver the majority of aerosol drugs efficiently?

4. Consider the hospitals through which you have rotated:

   a. What device(s) do they use to humidify the gas coming from the mechanical ventilators?

   b. How do they decide which device to use?

5. You receive an order to administer albuterol and ipratropium to a patient with a tracheostomy tube. Describe some ways you could do this.

CHAPTER 22

Hyperinflation Therapy

INTRODUCTION

Pulmonary atelectasis is a condition characterized by areas of the lung that have collapsed. Although atelectasis is generally associated with upper abdominal and thoracic surgery, it can occur anytime when lung expansion is limited. Factors that predispose a patient to atelectasis are obesity, general anesthesia, and preexisting pulmonary disease. Atelectasis can result from three mechanisms that may act independently or in combination: inadequate lung distending forces, airway obstruction, and loss of pulmonary surfactant.

Patients must be assessed for the presence of any of the risk factors prior to surgery, before procedures that require sedation, or before procedures that result in extended periods of immobilization. The RT must also assess when possible therapy should begin preoperatively when risk factors are present. Appropriate therapy should continue postoperatively until the patient is ambulating. The patient's condition and effectiveness of the treatment plan must be assessed often and therapy adjusted accordingly.

Discussion Activities and Questions

1. List at least two conditions that can cause atelectasis to occur.

2. What is the relationship between elastic recoil, pleural pressure, and lung expansion?

3. Explain the significance and implications of the Sugarloaf Conference.

4. What safeguards are built into the lung that provide collateral ventilation?

5. Describe the spontaneous breathing pattern that is most effective in minimizing or reversing atelectasis.

6. Describe the basic difference between flow-dependent and volume displacement incentive spirometers.

7. Explain the potential benefits of EPAP therapy.

8. Describe the proper procedure for IPPB.

REVIEW

True or False

—— 1. Atelectasis can contribute to the development of pneumonia.

—— 2. A tension pneumothorax can cause obstructive atelectasis.

—— 3. The Sugarloaf Conference generally concluded that the clinical evidence could not support the widespread use of IPPB.

—— 4. Glossopharyngeal breathing is a very useful technique for patients with COPD.

—— 5. Sustained maximal inflation and incentive spirometry are the same breathing technique.

—— 6. A volume displacement incentive spirometer of 4 L is most useful for pediatric patients.

—— 7. During EPAP therapy, the patient exhales against a threshold resistor.

—— 8. EPAP therapy can be used in conjunction with aerosol therapy.

—— 9. Passive IPPB therapy appears to result in the greatest post-treatment inspiratory capacity.

—— 10. IPPB therapy can be used with children.

Multiple Choice

1. A hyperinflation maneuver emphasizes inflation to which of the following?

   a. total lung capacity
   b. inspiratory capacity
   c. vital capacity
   d. functional residual capacity

2. Which of the following is the primary purpose of hyperinflation therapy?

   a. facilitate secretion removal
   b. facilitate bronchodilation
   c. treat hypoxemia
   d. prevention and treatment of atelectasis

3. You are asked to coach and encourage deep breathing for a patient who had upper abdominal surgery 12 hours ago. Which of the following is most important to determine prior to approaching the patient?

   a. recent vital signs
   b. time of last pain medication
   c. oxygenation status
   d. level of education

4. An 82-year-old female with severe dementia is admitted to the hospital with pneumonia and bilateral atelectasis. It is thought that she would benefit from hyperinflation therapy. Which of the following would be best for this patient?

   a. IPPB
   b. incentive spirometry
   c. directed cough
   d. glossopharyngeal breathing

5. If a patient does not decrease his or her respiratory rate during an IPPB treatment, which of the following side effects is most likely to occur?

   a. tachycardia
   b. hypoxemia
   c. hyperventilation
   d. tension pneumothorax

Lab Activities

1. Consider the hospitals through which you have rotated:

   a. What equipment do they have for hyperinflation therapy?

   b. How often is this therapy administered?

2. With regard to intermittent CPAP therapy:

   a. What equipment would you need to set this up?

   b. How would you determine the appropriate flow and FiO_2?

   c. How would you control the flow and FiO_2?

CHAPTER 23

Pulmonary Hygiene and Chest Physical Therapy

INTRODUCTION

Under normal conditions, pulmonary hygiene is on-going, and individuals are generally unaware of the processes involved. When chronic or debilitating illnesses develop, patients often need assistance to maintain pulmonary hygiene, ranging from education and encouragement to complex devices and regimens.

The chapter reviewed a number of techniques and devices that are used to promote the removal of retained secretions and to reduce the likelihood of progressive worsening of pulmonary function. Proper nutrition and fluid balance, as well as the incorporation of physical conditioning into the care plan, should not be neglected. The use of pharmacologic agents to improve air distribution and alter the physical characteristics of mucus must also be considered when appropriate. Additionally, the caregiver must be prepared to remove secretions by performing tracheal aspiration when necessary.

The selection of therapy modalities and development of a care plan must be based on the nature of the problems being addressed, the patient's ability or desire to comply with proposed regimens, and the complexity of equipment and associated expenses.

Discussion Activities and Questions

1. Describe the principal components of the mucociliary escalator.

2. Describe the four phases of a cough.

3. List three factors that might alter the effectiveness of coughing.

4. What is the significance of the MEP?

5. You are seeing a patient who has undergone a bowel resection. Assessment reveals that she now has serious secretion retention. List at least three techniques you can employ to help this patient effectively remove secretions.

6. Describe how you would teach a patient diaphragmatic breathing.

7. Describe the position for draining the apical segment of the right lower lobe.

8. Describe the techniques of percussion and vibration.

9. List and describe two devices that employ vibratory positive expiratory pressure therapy.

10. Describe the function of high-frequency chest wall oscillation.

REVIEW

True or False

_____ 1. Among other things, respiratory mucus contains glycoproteins.

_____ 2. In the mucociliary system, the sol layer is more viscous than the gel layer.

_____ 3. Dehydration can disrupt normal ciliary function.

_____ 4. Deep breathing and variations in breathing pattern can contribute to secretion retention.

_____ 5. Peak cough flows of greater than 200 Lpm may be necessary to prevent upper respiratory tract infections.

_____ 6. CPT can be safely performed on young children.

_____ 7. Active cycle of breathing cannot be used with young children.

_____ 8. PEP therapy helps to splint the airways.

_____ 9. High-frequency chest wall oscillation is also referred to as internal oscillation of the chest.

_____ 10. The device for intrapulmonary percussive ventilation therapy is also capable of delivering a medicated aerosol.

Multiple Choice

1. Mucostasis is a frequent complication of which of the following diseases?

   a. sarcoidosis
   b. myasthenia gravis
   c. idiopathic pulmonary fibrosis
   d. pneumonia

2. Which of the following is a normal mechanism that is most likely to assist with the removal of mucus?

   a. narrowing of the airways during exhalation
   b. dehydration of mucus
   c. application of negative pressure to the airway
   d. increasing the diameter of the airways during inhalation

3. Which of the following is a disease most likely to require CPT?

   a. pneumonia

   b. asthma

   c. cystic fibrosis

   d. silicosis

4. Which of the following are factors that can hinder the body's ability to clear mucus from the lung?

       1. shallow breathing
       2. cigarette smoking
       3. presence of artificial airway
       4. underhumidification

   a. 1, 2

   b. 1, 2, 3, 4

   c. 1, 3

   d. 2, 3, 4

5. Which of the following pulmonary function parameters is most likely to predict that a patient will have an ineffective cough?

   a. decreased FEF_{25-75}

   b. decreased FEV_1

   c. decreased FVC

   d. decreased FRC

6. How many different postural drainage positions are employed to assist in the drainage of secretions?

   a. 6

   b. 7

   c. 8

   d. 9

7. For which of the following patients should you exercise extreme caution when applying percussion and vibration?

   a. 10-year-old with cystic fibrosis

   b. 65-year-old with pneumonia and congestive heart failure

   c. 70-year-old with pneumonia who had a stroke 6 months ago

   d. 74-year-old with pneumonia and osteoporosis

8. Which of the following patients is most likely to benefit from the Philips Respironics Cough Assist device?

   a. C4 quadriplegic

   b. stage III COPD

   c. cystic fibrosis

   d. idiopathic pulmonary fibrosis

9. Continuous lateral rotation therapy provides a mechanical turning of the body a minimum of how many degrees?

   a. 40

   b. 45

   c. 50

   d. 60

10. Which of the following techniques would be best to use on a 42-year-old obtunded post-stroke patient with pneumonia secondary to secretion retention?

   a. HFCWO

   b. Acapella®

   c. autogenic drainage

   d. PDPV

Lab Activities

1. Based on your experience both as a trained observer and as a person who has experience coughing:

   a. Do you believe you can determine the adequacy of the cough?

   b. What assessment criteria do you use?

2. Consider the hospitals through which you have rotated:

   a. What techniques and equipment have the RTs used for CPT?

   b. What kinds of patients typically have received CPT?

Airway Management

INTRODUCTION

Airway management is one of the areas of care that respiratory therapists perform so routinely that they sometimes overlook its importance. With the artificial airways, emergency airway adjuncts, airway adjuncts, and speech aids for tracheostomy patients, as well as suctioning capabilities, all constantly improving, RTs have the tools to be ever more effective with airway management. Their duty is to be the most informed member of the health-care team and match the appropriate patient with the most effective modalities. Numerous devices and techniques have not been changed significantly since they were introduced to clinical practice. The reason is that they are useful as introduced and they blend in with the new technologies to provide the tools necessary for airway management.

Discussion Activities and Questions

1. What is the goal of airway management?

2. Describe the differences between the Berman and the Guedel airways.

3. List and describe at least three methods for verifying proper placement of the endotracheal tube.

4. What is the purpose of a lighted stylet?

5. List three advantages of nasotracheal intubation, as opposed to orotracheal intubation.

6. What are the principal differences between the LMA and the Combitube airway?

7. List at least three advantages of a tracheostomy over an endotracheal tube.

8. What are the advantages of using a foam-filled cuff on a tracheostomy tube?

9. Compare the three methods of monitoring cuff pressures.

10. List three characteristics of a good suction catheter.

REVIEW

True or False

_____ 1. When a person is experiencing partial airway obstruction, he or she is incapable of producing sound.

_____ 2. During an intubation, if the ET tube is inserted too far, it will most likely go into the right main-stem bronchus.

_____ 3. A gum elastic bougie can be used to facilitate blind intubation.

_____ 4. Inadvertent extubation is more common with nasal intubation.

_____ 5. On the Cormack and Lahane scale, a grade of 1 would indicate that the intubation will be more difficult.

_____ 6. A cricothyrotomy is generally used to establish an emergency airway.

_____ 7. One problem that occurs with a mature tracheostomy stoma is increased airway resistance.

_____ 8. The Passy-Muir speaking valve cannot be used with fenestrated tracheostomy tubes.

_____ 9. An undersized tracheostomy tube will generally require high cuff pressures.

_____ 10. Suction catheters must be less than one-quarter the diameter of the artificial airway being suctioned.

Multiple Choice

1. Which of the following patients is most likely to benefit from an artificial airway?

   a. asthma exacerbation
   b. COPD exacerbation
   c. failure secondary to idiopathic pulmonary fibrosis
   d. progressive Guillain-Barré syndrome

2. You are about to intubate a patient. What is the maximum number of seconds you can allow for the attempt before you stop and reoxygenate the patient?

   a. 20
   b. 30
   c. 40
   d. 60

3. You need to intubate an 8-month-old who has presented to the ED in respiratory failure. What is the best endotracheal tube to use?

   a. 3.0–3.5 uncuffed
   b. 3.5–4.5 uncuffed
   c. 4.5–5.5 uncuffed
   d. 5.5–6.5 uncuffed

4. Immediately after extubating a patient, you note mild respiratory distress and inspiratory stridor. Which of the following is the best course of action to take at this time?

   a. Administer racemic epinephrine via small-volume nebulizer.
   b. Administer oxygen via nonrebreathing mask.
   c. Administer levalbuterol via small-volume nebulizer.
   d. Reintubate.

5. Which of the following is the material most commonly used to make tracheostomy tubes?

   a. rubber
   b. silicone
   c. PVC
   d. Teflon

6. Which of the following conditions may be indications for the use of special speech aids in patients with tracheostomy tubes?

   1. tracheomalacia
   2. head trauma
   3. quadriplegia
   4. mild tracheal stenosis

   a. 1, 2, 3, 4
   b. 1, 3
   c. 2, 3, 4
   d. 3, 4

7. Upon measuring a patient's cuff pressure with a cuff manometer, you note that the pressure reads 22 mm Hg. What effect will this have on circulation in the tracheal wall?

   a. reduced lymphatic flow only
   b. reduced venous flow
   c. reduced arterial flow
   d. no effect

8. When suctioning a patient with an endotracheal tube, you should advance the catheter until which of the following?

   a. resistance is felt
   b. the patient starts to cough
   c. at least 10 cm
   d. the whistle tip is even with the tube opening

Lab Activities

1. Think about the hospitals through which you have rotated:

   a. What kinds of emergency airways (excluding endotracheal and tracheostomy tubes) do they have available?

   b. How are these used? How often?

2. Recall patients you have seen at various hospitals who have had ET tubes inserted:

    a. Typically, how have these tubes been secured?

    b. In your opinion, what is the best way to secure an endotracheal tube?

3. Using various Internet sources, find videos of the following procedures:

    a. fiberoptic intubation

    b. percutaneous tracheotomy

    c. cricothyrotomy

    d. tracheostomy care

4. In the health-care facilities through which you have rotated:

    a. Who does the routine tracheostomy care?

    b. How often is it done?

    c. Who does the tracheostomy tube changes?

    d. How often are tube changes done?

Physiological Effects of Mechanical Ventilation

INTRODUCTION

Mechanically ventilated patients are at risk for a number of complications associated with the physiological effects of positive pressure ventilation. To effectively provide positive pressure ventilation while alleviating the potential hazards of mechanical ventilation, the respiratory therapist needs to understand the physiological changes that result from mechanical ventilation. Early recognition of the potential effects enables the therapist to prevent further complications.

Discussion Activities and Questions

1. Explain the goals of negative and positive pressure ventilation in relation to transpulmonary pressure.

2. List the three methods by which artificial mechanical ventilation can be administered.

3. List three factors that can cause an increase in airway resistance.

4. Explain the difference between dynamic and static compliance.

5. List the two strategy limbs in oxygen and PEEP titration that have been found acceptable in the treatment of a patient who has acute lung injury or acute respiratory distress syndrome.

6. Explain what effect a decreased lung compliance can have on time constants.

7. List three methods that can be used to decrease plateau pressures.

8. Explain some of the differences between negative and positive pressure ventilation.

9. Explain some of the differences between positive pressure and high-frequency ventilation.

10. List three complications that can occur from mechanical ventilation.

REVIEW

True or False

—— 1. Negative pressure ventilation is the only method that uses active exhalation.

—— 2. Decreasing the tidal volume can help decrease plateau pressure.

—— 3. Positive pressure ventilation can cause an increase in cardiac output.

—— 4. High mean airway pressures can impede blood flow to the brain.

—— 5. Hyperoxia-related injuries occur when patients are exposed to high levels of oxygen for prolonged periods of time.

—— 6. Transairway pressure reflects the pressure difference between the mouth and the chest wall.

—— 7. High-frequency ventilation mimics normal respirations.

—— 8. "Lung compliance" refers to the change in flow over the change in pressure.

—— 9. Dynamic compliance measures changes in volume and pressure in the nonelastic airways.

—— 10. It is necessary to obtain a static lung hold when calculating dynamic compliance.

Multiple Choice

1. All of the following are complications of mechanical ventilation except:

   a. increased cardiac output
   b. volutrauma
   c. barotraumas
   d. decreased cerebral perfusion

2. The normal airway resistance of a nonintubated patient is:

   a. 1.2–3.2 cmH_2O/L/sec
   b. 4–5 mm Hg
   c. 0.6–2.4 cmH_2O/L/sec
   d. 40–60 cmH_2O

3. How many time constants should fill approximately 98% of a lung unit?

   a. 1
   b. 3
   c. 5
   d. 4

4. To prevent barotrauma, plateau pressure should be:

   a. <20 cmH_2O
   b. >30 cmH_2O
   c. <50 cmH_2O
   d. <30 cmH_2O

5. Target tidal volumes for an adult patient with ARDS or acute lung injury should be in what range?

   a. 4–8 mL/kg ideal body weight
   b. 10–15 mL/kg ideal body weight

   c. 20–30 mL/kg ideal body weight
   d. 40–60 mL/kg ideal body weight

Lab Activities

1. When initiating mechanical ventilation on a patient, what parameters would you want to assess to determine the patient's static and dynamic compliance?

2. Your ventilated patient has developed an increased airway resistance. What steps can you take to reduce the resistance?

3. Discuss the two limbed oxygen/PEEP titration strategies. Which strategy do you believe could be more beneficial to a patient who has ARDS?

4. When ventilating a patient who has asthma, which compliance (dynamic, static) would you want to measure and why?

5. Discuss the major differences between barotrauma and volutrauma. Is one condition more important than the other? Explain.

Initiation, Monitoring, and Discontinuing Mechanical Ventilation

INTRODUCTION

The initiation and management of a patient on mechanical ventilation require a thorough understanding of the function of various ventilator modes and how changes in the patient's compliance and resistance affect gas delivery. Respiratory therapists need to be able to determine the primary control variable during the inspiratory phase to make sense of the ventilator manufacturer's mode terminology. For example, it's important to clarify what is actually meant by the term "spontaneous breathing" when it is used to describe any given mode. Knowledge of how a specific ventilator breath is triggered, limited, and cycled, coupled with basic cardiopulmonary physiology, provides the foundation for appropriate patient application, management, and subsequent discontinuation of mechanical ventilation.

Discussion Activities and Questions

1. List some of the reasons for initiating mechanical ventilation.

2. Using what you have learned from this chapter, explain what ventilatory failure is.

3. Using what you have learned from this chapter, explain what oxygenation failure is.

4. Explain what extracorporeal membrane oxygenation (ECMO) is and how it benefits the patient.

5. Explain how PEEP could increase FRC.

6. List some methods of alveolar recruitment.

7. Define "impending ventilatory failure." Does it differ from acute ventilatory failure?

8. List some of the guidelines for initiation of mechanical ventilation.

9. Explain how a ventilator check is performed.

10. How was compliance calculated on older-model ventilators?

REVIEW

True or False

_____ 1. Oxygenation failure is not an indication for initiating mechanical ventilation.

_____ 2. Acute ventilatory failure is an indication for initiating mechanical ventilation.

_____ 3. HMEs should be removed when an aerosol treatment is delivered through the ventilator.

_____ 4. Ventilator-associated pneumonia (VAP) usually develops within 30 minutes of intubation.

_____ 5. Alveolar recruitment is the reopening of collapsed alveoli.

_____ 6. Bilevel ventilation allows for spontaneous breathing.

_____ 7. Independent lung ventilation utilizes a double lumen-end tracheal tube as well as two ventilators.

_____ 8. Increasing PEEP is generally the best method for increasing mean airway pressure.

_____ 9. Increasing PEEP can increase the pulmonary vascular resistance (PRV) and decrease the blood pressure gradient for venous return to the heart.

Multiple Choice

1. PEEP can impair the function of the:

   a. brain
   b. lungs
   c. kidneys
   d. all of the above

2. Barotrauma is another type of ventilator-associated lung injury that is more closely related to _____ than to _____.

   a. absolute airway pressure, regional lung distention
   b. regional lung distention, absolute airway pressure
   c. airway pressure, airway mean
   d. airway mean, regional lung distention

3. AARC guidelines for removing an endotracheal tube recommend a negative inspiratory force of:

   a. >30 cmH$_2$O
   b. < 20 cmH$_2$O
   c. 15 cmH$_2$O
   d. >8 cmH$_2$O

4. All extubations should be performed by clinicians who are capable of:

   a. walking
   b. breathing
   c. working
   d. providing mask and bag ventilation

5. The screening criteria that may be included in an extubation protocol are:

   a. P/F > 150

   b. PEEP < 5

   c. NIF > 20

   d. all of the above

Lab Activities

For this section, get help from the instructor.

1. Using a test lung attached to a ventilator on Assist Control setting, observe and record the following parameters: PIP, PEEP, plateau pressure, mean airway pressure, compliance, and airway resistance. Adjust the test lung for more or less resistance. How do these numbers change?

2. Using a test lung attached to a ventilator on Pressure Control setting, observe and record the following parameters: PIP, PEEP, plateau pressure, mean airway pressure, compliance, inspiratory time, I:E ratio, and airway resistance. Adjust the test lung for more or less resistance. How do these numbers change?

3. Place the ventilator on Bilevel and adjust the settings to Phigh and Plow and Thigh and Tlow.

4. Take the test lung and place the ventilator on different modes, such as CPAP and SIMV.

5. Practice setting the alarms as well as the apnea parameters on the ventilator. Discuss what factors could cause the alarms to sound, as well as what could make the ventilator go into apnea settings.

CHAPTER 27

Mechanics and Modes of Mechanical Ventilation

INTRODUCTION

Currently available mechanical ventilators that are designed for use in critical care have ventilator graphic displays (or, at a minimum, options to include ventilator graphics). Ventilator graphics have provided the respiratory therapist with a clinically significant tool for managing patient-ventilator interactions, monitoring pulmonary mechanics, and detecting clinically significant issues with the ventilator system.

Mastering the interpretation of ventilator graphics can be challenging for the respiratory therapist, but understanding ventilator graphics is an important element in the improvement of patient care in critical care and other patient care areas.

This chapter provides a fundamental approach to understanding the information that ventilator graphics provide and the analysis of that information. Some of the commonly observed abnormal patterns have been discussed in this chapter. However, not every clinical situation and/or every available ventilator could be included. Respiratory therapists are challenged to continue to improve their understanding and utilize ventilator graphics as a tool to enhance patient care and management of patient-ventilator interactions. Follow-up suggested readings are included at the end of the chapter, and manufacturers' representatives and Web sites can provide equipment-specific information. Experienced colleagues can also be a valuable resource by sharing their accumulated knowledge.

Discussion Activities and Questions

1. List the three primary variables that are assessed with waveforms.

2. Calculate total cycle time (TCT) if the ventilator is set for a respiratory rate of 8 breaths per minute with an inspiratory time of 1 second. (60 sec/RR = TCT).

3. Calculate TCT if the ventilator is set for a respiratory rate of 10 breaths per minute with an inspiratory time of 1 second.

4. Define "positive end expiratory pressure."

5. Explain some of the major differences between volume ventilation and pressure ventilation.

6. Explain some of the different modes of ventilation available in volume ventilation.

7. Explain the different modes of ventilation available in pressure ventilation.

8. Identify the inspiratory and expiratory phases from the waveforms in the following figure.

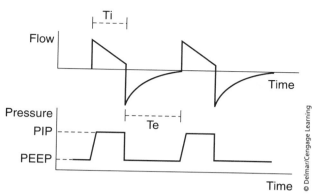

9. Using the second waveform in the following figure, identify the PIP and the PEEP.

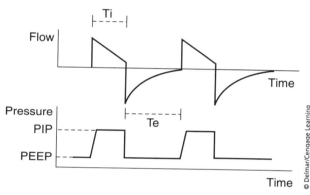

10. Give a brief description of each of the major waveforms (square, decelerating, sine, etc.).

REVIEW

True or False

_____ 1. Ventilator graphics has provided the respiratory therapist with a clinically significant tool for managing patient-ventilator interactions, monitoring pulmonary mechanics, and detecting clinically significant issues with the ventilator system.

_____ 2. The shape of the flow-volume loop (FVL) can look different depending on the mode set on the ventilator and whether pressure or volume ventilation is being used.

_____ 3. A volume pressure loop that shifts to the right is indicative of stiff lungs.

_____ 4. An I:E ratio of 1:3 would be considered an inverse ratio.

_____ 5. A sensitivity setting where the patient has to make a great effort to trigger a breath is called autocycling.

_____ 6. Auto-PEEP can have a negative impact on triggering.

_____ 7. Mean airway pressure (MAP) is the average pressure occurring in the airway during the complete respiratory cycle.

_____ 8. The I:E ratio is simply a proportion of the inspiratory and expiratory time in a respiratory cycle.

_____ 9. Resistance consists of frictional forces associated with ventilation due to the anatomical structure of conduit airways and the resistance to gas flow through the airways, and the viscous resistance of the lungs and the adjacent tissues and organs as the lungs expand and contract.

_____ 10. RAW stands for "airways resistance."

Multiple Choice

1. The _____ scalar waveform is generated by a constant flow rate throughout inspiration. The waveform can also be referred to as a rectangular or constant flow rate wave.

   a. accelerating
   b. sinusoidal

   c. square
   d. decelerating

2. The _____ waveform is generated by flow that increases to a peak and then decreases. At times only half of this curve may be present.

   a. accelerating
   b. sinusoidal

   c. square
   d. decelerating

3. The _____ waveform is generated by flow that begins with a low level and then increases throughout inspiration. This waveform has also been called an ascending waveform.

   a. accelerating
   b. sinusoidal

   c. square
   d. decelerating

4. The _____ waveform is generated by flow that begins at a low level and then increases gradually throughout inspiration.

   a. accelerating
   b. rise

   c. square
   d. decelerating

5. The _____ waveform is generated by flow that begins at peak and decreases in a linear manner until the end of inspiration. This waveform is also known as a descending waveform.

   a. accelerating
   b. sinusoidal

   c. square
   d. decelerating

Lab Activities

1. Calculate the total cycle time in 60 seconds for each respiratory rate listed in the following table.

Time	Respiratory Rate	TCT
60 sec	60	1
60 sec	30	
60 sec	20	
60 sec	15	
60 sec	12	
60 sec	10	
60 sec	6	

2. Identify the first, second, and third wave graphics in the following figure. Which one is volume, which one is pressure, and which one is flow?

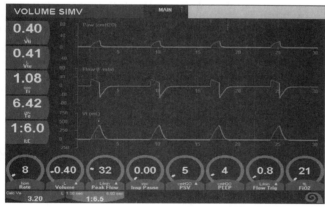

Courtesy of CareFusion

3. Name the flow waveform in the following figure. What type of waveform is this? Sinusoidal waveform, accelerating waveform, decelerating waveform, or square waveform?

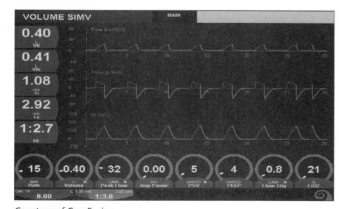

Courtesy of CareFusion

CHAPTER **2 8**

Noninvasive Mechanical Ventilation

INTRODUCTION

Although noninvasive ventilation is not new, the technology associated with noninvasive positive pressure ventilation (NPPV) has improved since the 1990s. In the acute care setting, NPPV may be an alternative to intubation and invasive ventilation in 75% of the patients with acute exacerbation of COPD. Long-term NPPV is an option for select patients with COPD who meet Medicare's coverage criteria. The use of negative pressure ventilation in the same patient population is not currently supported by the results of clinical trials, but may be useful in patients unable to tolerate mask ventilation. Finally, CPAP or NPPV application represents the current standard of care in cases of acute cardiogenic pulmonary edema.

Discussion Activities and Questions

1. List some of the goals of NPPV.

2. List the criteria for using NPPV.

3. List some of the benefits of using NPPV.

4. Explain some of the differences between NPPV and invasive ventilation.

5. List the relative contraindications for using NPPV.

6. List the absolute contraindications for using NPPV.

7. List all the different types of NPPV. How do these types differ from each other?

8. List the initial settings used for NPPV (BIPAP).

9. Explain the different settings for NPPV (BIPAP) and their function.

10. Explain how IPAP and EPAP are used in BIPAP.

11. Explain the difference between NPPV (BIPAP) and CPAP.

REVIEW

True or False

_____ 1. NPPV is not indicated for respiratory failure.

_____ 2. The patient-ventilator interface in NPPV is usually an endotracheal tube.

_____ 3. It may take up to 20 hours for some patients to respond to NPPV.

_____ 4. CPAP breathing was used as a method of delivering oxygen to pilots flying at high altitudes during World War II.

_____ 5. Only MDIs can be used in NPPV.

_____ 6. Noninvasive ventilation is contraindicated in the presence of respiratory muscle fatigue.

_____ 7. A common complaint with NPPV is skin breakdown on patients.

_____ 8. Patients with facial burns can use NPPV (BIPAP).

_____ 9. Patients who are hemodynamically unstable on BIPAP (NPPV) should continue on BIPAP.

_____ 10. If patients need airway protection, they can receive BIPAP (NPPV).

Multiple Choice

1. What is the goal of using NPPV?

   a. decrease the flow to the patient
   b. improve on gas exchange
   c. decrease the I:E only
   d. decrease the oxygen

2. When placing a patient on BIPAP (NPPV), what is the purpose of IPAP and EPAP?

   a. improve gas exchange
   b. decrease the CO_2 arterial blood gas levels
   c. deliver a tidal volume
   d. all of the above

3. Increasing only the IPAP setting on BIPAP will:

   a. decrease the flow
   b. increase the tidal volume
   c. decrease the CO_2
   d. both b and c

4. CPAP can help reduce the intubation rate for patients with:

   a. facial burns
   b. pulmonary edema
   c. respiratory arrest
   d. ARDS

5. Relative complications of BIPAP include:

   a. COPD
   b. ARDS
   c. extreme anxiety
   d. both b and c

Lab Activities

1. Discuss the purpose of NPPV and how it can prevent patients from being placed on invasive ventilation.

2. Explain the differences between the different types of NPPV.

3. Discuss the initial settings for BIPAP (NPPV). What adjustments could you make to reduce a patient's P_aCO_2 level? What could be done to improve oxygenation?

4. Discuss the various settings and their functions in BIPAP (NPPV) therapy.

5. Explain what the major difference is between the BIPAP (NPPV) and the Pulmo-Wrap.

Levels of Care Delivery

Neonatal and Pediatric Respiratory Care

INTRODUCTION

Respiratory care of the pediatric patient presents clinicians with unique challenges. An understanding of the diseases and pathologies related to infants and children is essential to craft effective respiratory care for this population. The size and complexity of some pediatric patients present special challenges when using technology in their treatment. Some techniques that work well in adult scenarios perform differently in these populations, such as oxygen delivery, aerosol delivery, mechanical ventilation, and airway management. Recently, certain practices have been exposed as ineffective or inefficient, including blow-by oxygen or aerosol delivery and the use of pneumatic (jet) nebulizers for the delivery of aerosolized medications.

Discussion Activities and Questions

1. Differentiate between a newborn and a pediatric patient.

2. Explain why air oxygen blenders are now being used more in labor and delivery rooms.

3. Explain how the fetus receives enriched oxygenated blood and nutrients in utero.

4. List two important circumstances during resuscitation of newborns.

5. Explain the Apgar scores and what five signs are evaluated by an Apgar score.

6. Explain when Apgar scores are typically assessed (at what time after delivery) by the respiratory therapist, nurse, or doctor participating in the resuscitation.

7. Explain what a pneumothorax is and what may happen if it is not treated.

8. List the three major types of shunting present in the newborn.

9. List at least three maternal factors that can lead to premature birth.

10. Explain the major role that the respiratory therapist has in reducing the risk of ROP.

REVIEW

True or False

_____ 1. Patients of all ages with a chronic disease who have been managed by pediatric subspecialists may still be seen by their pediatric subspecialists.

_____ 2. Approach to resuscitation would include initial resuscitation with 30–40% oxygen for very preterm infants using targeted SpO_2 values.

_____ 3. From birth to 4 weeks old is the definition of a neonate.

_____ 4. U.S. hospitals receive about 30 million emergency visits from the population under 18 years of age.

_____ 5. More than one in eight babies are born prematurely each year in the United States.

_____ 6. In utero, the fetal requirements for oxygen and nutrients are supplied by the oxygenated blood flowing from the placenta to the fetus.

_____ 7. During the resuscitation of newborns, there are two important circumstances in which special considerations are required.

_____ 8. Dr. Virginia Apgar created the method of assessing the cardiorespiratory status of infants at delivery and of assessing the effectiveness of resuscitation efforts.

_____ 9. One of the most common causes of vision loss in childhood is retinopathy of prematurity.

_____ 10. Since 1981, the rate of premature births in the United States has increased by 31%.

Multiple Choice

1. Which of the following statements concerning congenital diaphragmatic hernia (CDH) is true?

    a. If large enough, the defect will allow abdominal contents to enter the chest cavity.
    b. A defect or hole can occur in the diaphragm during intrauterine lung development.
    c. The abdominal structures can press on a developing lung and hinder lung growth.
    d. All of the above.

2. One misconception about neonatal and pediatric practice is which of the following?

    a. Children are small adults and neonates are merely smaller pediatric patients.
    b. They are harder or more demanding.
    c. No additional training is required for a pediatric or neonatal RT.
    d. Both a and b.

3. When the fetus is in utero, the placenta provides _____ for the fetus.

    a. CO_2-enriched blood
    b. oxygen-enriched blood

    c. nutrients
    d. both b and c

4. What two circumstances raise special considerations and concerns during the resuscitation of newborns?

    a. meconium
    b. full-term baby

    c. diaphragmatic hernia
    d. both a and c

5. Infants are considered premature if they are born under _____ weeks estimated gestational age (EGA).

    a. 42
    b. 37

    c. 54
    d. 69

Lab Activities

1. Discuss some of the misconceptions surrounding the care of neonates and pediatric patients.

2. Discuss the fetal circulatory pathway and how it differs in utero from after delivery.

3. Discuss some of the methods that may be employed to avoid heat loss in newborns.

4. Explain what efforts would be made regarding a patient born with meconium.

5. Discuss some of the key factors in performing a respiratory assessment of a pediatric patient.

C H A P T E R **3 0**

Geriatric Applications

INTRODUCTION

In 2002, a document titled "Ten Reasons Why America Is Not Ready for the Coming Age Boom" was published by the Alliance for Aging Research. Their statistics are compelling, their message even more so. Despite increased numbers of older adult patients, physicians trained in geriatrics will be woefully lacking. The same goes for allied health professionals; there will be more older patients, but fewer therapists (occupational therapy, physical therapy, respiratory therapy) will be trained in bedside geriatric care. The approaching and very real geriatric gap has the potential to overwhelm the health-care system.

It does not have to be that way. The graying of America will offer superior job security to those who are competent in the skills and knowledge required to care for the aging population. The aged patient will challenge the therapist to look beyond the obvious answers. Therapists will need to use all their clinical skills, senses, intuition, reasoning, and common sense to provide safe and competent care. Change can take place only if there is a determined effort to turn the corner and embrace geriatric educational initiatives. The older adult patient population will be available; the time to train is now.

Discussion Activities and Questions

1. What are the implications of an aging minority population?

2. What is the principal difference between Medicare Part A and Part B?

3. Give at least three reasons why physical evaluation of an older person might take more time.

4. List at least four chronic diseases often reported by older adults.

5. What is the difference between ADLS and IADLS?

6. List at least two symptoms of hearing loss.

7. List at least three ways to help a patient who has a hearing impairment.

8. List at least three signs of malnutrition in elderly patients.

9. List at least three factors that can decrease dexterity in the elderly.

10. List four factors that contribute to adverse drug reactions and noncompliance with medication regimes.

Thought Questions

1. Think about people you know who are over the age of 85. Are they basically healthy? What health issues (either major or minor) have they experienced?

2. Think about patients you have seen in the clinical setting. Did their chronological age match their appearance? If not, what factors might account for the discrepancy?

3. Consider some elderly people you know. Evaluate their ability to perform ADLs and IADLs.

4. You have a home care patient who uses oxygen via nasal cannula attached to an oxygen concentrator. He also uses multiple inhalers. He has some vision impairment. Suggest some ways the patient can accommodate this impairment.

5. You are asked to see an 80-year-old female in her home because she has been put on oxygen. In doing an environmental assessment, list at least seven things you would look for. How would you help to correct any deficiencies?

6. Using the AARC or a similar resource, determine the cost of the following inhalers: Advair 250/50, Spiriva, albuterol (or ProAir).

7. Examine the medical record of at least one elderly patient. Based on what you see in the record, do you believe the patient will have problems, either during the hospital stay or upon discharge? If so, is there anything you can do to help the patient minimize these problems?

REVIEW

True or False

——— 1. Women have a longer life expectancy than men.

——— 2. People over the age of 85 cannot be eligible for both Medicare and Medicaid.

——— 3. Total body water is most likely to increase as we age.

——— 4. Chronological age is a good indicator of physiological age.

——— 5. Older adults may have atypical presentations of diseases.

——— 6. People with cataracts generally become more sensitive to light.

——— 7. In general, high-pitched tones are easier to hear than low-pitched tones.

——— 8. The Clock Drawing Test is an element used in cognitive assessment.

——— 9. Polypharmacy never does harm to patients.

——— 10. When teaching a new technique, ask the patient for a return demonstration.

Multiple Choice

1. Approximately what percent of acute care patients are over the age of 65?

    a. 50
    b. 60
    c. 70
    d. 80

2. All of the following are core elements of a CGA except:

    a. functional assessment
    b. cognitive assessment
    c. financial assessment
    d. physical assessment

3. You are attempting to teach a 70-year-old male with COPD the proper way to use a metered-dose inhaler. You begin by demonstrating the proper method; however, the patient seems to have problems following the demonstration. Which of the following chronic problems is the most likely cause?

    a. arthritis
    b. cataracts
    c. diabetes
    d. macular degeneration

4. You are creating a brochure for patients who might have visual disorders. Which of the following would it be best not to use?

    a. orange
    b. green
    c. yellow
    d. red

5. You are attempting to review inhaler instructions with a patient who has Alzheimer's disease. The patient may have trouble complying because of which of the following?

    a. memory deficit
    b. poor comprehension
    c. limited hand-eye coordination
    d. persistent tremor

Emergency Respiratory Care

INTRODUCTION

In dealing with a patient emergency, the critical priorities are circulation, airway, and breathing. The new priority in the pulseless patient is compressions. The sequence depends on available resources. If someone is unconscious and unresponsive and the therapist is alone with an AED at hand, he should call 911, perform 5 cycles of 30 compressions and 2 breaths, then attach the AED and evaluate the rhythm and shock as appropriate. If there are two rescuers, one calls 911 and retrieves the AED on the way back from calling 911; the other initiates CPR with compressions. If there are three rescuers, one calls 911, one obtains and applies the AED, and the third begins CPR—and so on.

Discussion Activities and Questions

1. What is meant by placing the patient in the recovery position?

2. What are some signs indicating that a person is choking?

3. List three risk factors for coronary artery disease.

4. What is the main difference between BLS and ACLS?

5. Compare monophasic with biphasic defibrillators.

6. Describe the function and importance of the scribe during a resuscitation effort.

7. Describe the process of cardioversion. What is the principal difference between cardioversion and defibrillation?

8. Compare and contrast manual defibrillators with automated external defibrillators. What are advantages of each?

9. List five risk factors that indicate a potential need for neonatal resuscitation.

10. Describe the procedure of and the equipment necessary for intubating an infant. How do these differ from procedures and equipment used for an adult?

REVIEW

True or False

_____ 1. Some form of pocket mask should be available in every hospital room.

_____ 2. The vast majority of adults who suffer cardiac arrest have asystole as their initial rhythm.

_____ 3. Once it is discovered that a patient being resuscitated has a valid DNR order, the resuscitation should stop.

_____ 4. A positive result for an EDD indicates that the ET tube is in the esophagus.

_____ 5. It is always very useful to obtain arterial blood gas data during a cardiac arrest.

_____ 6. Defibrillation poses no risk to the operator or the resuscitation team.

_____ 7. The normal values for vital signs are about the same for infants as for adults.

_____ 8. Epinephrine is the drug that should be given first to a young child with symptomatic bradycardia.

_____ 9. Injury is the leading cause of death in children.

_____ 10. The combitube is designed to be inserted into the trachea.

Multiple Choice

1. Which of the following is considered a shockable rhythm?

   a. ventricular fibrillation
   b. asystole
   c. supraventricular tachycardia
   d. pulseless electrical activity

2. You are participating in the resuscitation of an elderly male who has experienced cardiac arrest. One rescuer is performing compressions while another is ventilating with a bag and mask. According to the 2010 guidelines from the American Heart Association, which of the following is the appropriate ratio of compressions to ventilation?

   a. 5:1
   b. 15:2
   c. 20:1
   d. 30:2

3. You are ventilating a 70-year-old female who has just been intubated following a successful resuscitation. You should provide breaths at what rate?

   a. 8–10 per minute
   b. 10–112 per minute
   c. 12–14 per minute
   d. 14–16 per minute

4. You are participating in the resuscitation of an adult cardiac arrest victim who is intubated. You attach a capnograph and monitor the $P_{ET}CO_2$ level. Which of the following $P_{ET}CO_2$ readings (in mm Hg) would indicate that circulation has not yet returned?

   a. 5

   b. 15

   c. 25

   d. 35

5. A patient presents in ventricular fibrillation. Which of the following drugs has shown the most benefit for increasing short-term survival in such patients?

   a. lidocaine

   b. atropine

   c. vasopressin

   d. amiodarone

6. You receive a stat call to the dialysis unit. Upon arrival, you note that a resuscitation effort is underway. The patient is an elderly male, who is lying supine on the floor. The monitor on the crash cart shows asystole. You are told that the patient was transported to dialysis after collapsing at home. He was apparently two days overdue for his dialysis appointment. Which of the following is the most likely cause of his asystole?

   a. hypoxia

   b. tension pneumothorax

   c. metabolic acidosis

   d. hyperkalemia

7. Which of the following is included in the initial treatment of a patient who presents with symptoms suggestive of myocardial ischemia?

   1. epinephrine
   2. morphine
   3. nitroglycerine
   4. atropine

   a. 1, 2, 4

   b. 1, 3

   c. 2, 3

   d. 2, 3, 4

8. A 2-year-old female is brought into the ED by her parents. She is unresponsive, is breathing shallowly, and has a weak pulse of 64 beats per minute. Her mother states that the child consumed an unknown quantity of oxycodone. Which of the following drugs should be administered as soon as possible?

   a. atropine

   b. epinephrine

   c. naloxone

   d. amiodarone

9. When ventilating a baby via bag and mask, which of the following is the simplest effective method of determining adequacy of ventilation?

   a. monitor $P_{ET}CO_2$

   b. listen to breath sounds

   c. observe chest rise

   d. measure tidal volume

10. Two attempts to insert a 5.0 cuffed ET tube in a 4-year-old who is in respiratory arrest have failed. Which of the following is the best alternative to try next?

    a. combitube

    b. LMA

    c. 4.0 uncuffed ET tube

    d. esophageal obturator

Lab Activities

1. Examine and compare the American Heart Association (AHA) 2005 guidelines for basic life support with the 2010 guidelines. In what significant way do they differ?

2. You are participating in the resuscitation of a 6-year-old male who was transported to the ED because of an accidental gunshot wound to the chest. After 20 minutes, the patient has not responded and there has been no spontaneous return of circulation. The physician directing the resuscitation effort declares that it is time to stop. How do you respond, and how do you feel about terminating the resuscitation?

3. Describe a cardiopulmonary arrest scenario that you observed or in which you participated. What was the outcome? How did you feel afterward?

4. Using the 2010 AHA guidelines, compare the resuscitation of a pulseless child to that of a pulseless adult. How are they same? How are they different?

CHAPTER 32

Managing Disasters: Respiratory Care in Mass Critical Care

INTRODUCTION

Disasters of any cause or size require a coordinated, prepared response if both the victims and the hospital are to survive. The NIMS and the hospital's ICS are the command and control elements of disaster response. Most disasters are Tier 1 and can be managed by prepared and drilled staff.

Standard Precautions, aerosol protection, and patient decontamination are more important in an MCI because of the many unknowns as the event unfolds. By establishing an early diagnosis and providing prompt, prepared aggressive care, the worst case can be forestalled. Accurate recordkeeping and the bagging and tagging of victims' personal possessions assist in the investigation that will follow the event.

The regular use of surge ventilators purchased by state or local governments for EMCC precludes or reduces training time. Among the ventilators purchased by state and local governments are the Viasys-Pulmonetics LTV 1200 and the Versamed iVent. Both are excellent volume-pressure-cycled ventilators with PEEP and oxygen options and an internal battery with about 1 hour's worth of use. However, both require annual servicing by company-certified technicians, mandatory battery recharge, and temperature-humidity-controlled storage.

The federal government's emergency National Strategic Stockpile Push Packs are 2-ton preloaded and prepositioned supply containers of medicines, equipment, and ventilators (no oxygen) that can be at a site within 12 hours of an emergency. Push Packs include the LP-10 and the Impact Eagle754 transport ventilators which, while easy to operate, still require in-service education that must be accomplished prior to a disaster of either natural causes or of human intent. The Eagle754 is a touch screen operation ventilator with internal battery (rechargeable) and compressor; it is therefore ideal for emergency situations. With an automatic pressure transducer, the 754 can support patients to an altitude of 25,000 feet. It is approved for use with adults and pediatric patients, including infants. Additionally, the Impact Eagle provides the intensive care level of mechanical ventilation that nurses, respiratory therapists, and intensivists have come to expect from their ventilators: alarms and graphics display.

Medicine and respiratory care in particular are constantly evolving sciences with new research and clinical experience that constantly broaden knowledge, skills, and pharmacologic treatment. They require respiratory therapists to maintain and update their knowledge and proficiency. The reader is strongly encouraged to confirm information contained in this chapter for updates, evidence-based studies, and clinical competencies.

Discussion Activities and Questions

1. What should hospitals have internally to support the National Incident Management System?

   Hospitals should have a hospital emergency incident command system.

2. List four examples of a worst-case disaster scenario.

   Loss of main oxygen supply, medical air supply, water supply or food supply.

3. What kinds of respiratory problems might be anticipated following an earthquake?

   Coccidioidomycosis infections, Hyperkalemia, Rhabdomyolysis, acute respiratory distress syndrome.

4. Describe the blast lung triad. *The lung blast triad of respiratory distress, hypoxia and a so-called butterfly or bat wing infiltrate appearance on chest x-ray has been described for over 30 yrs in medical literature. Meanwhile, the severity of the BLI can be categorized by P/F ratio, chest x-ray, and the presence or absence of a bronchopleural fistula. Signs & symptoms: Tachypnea, Dyspnea, cyanosis, Hemoptysis, decreased consciousness, decreased breath sounds w/ or w/out crackles.*

5. Describe the precautions necessary if a patient with a case of smallpox presents in the ED.

   Standard droplet precautions would need to be taken and we may treat the patient with antiviral agents like ribavirin and cidofovir in an aerosol therapy.

6. What is the classic triad of botulinum intoxication? *Symmetrical, descending paralysis with bulbar palsies of (the so-called 4 Ds): diplopia, dysarthria, dysphonia and dysphagia*
   * *an afebrile patient*
   * *Clear sensorium*

7. What is the role of the respiratory therapist in dealing with a bioterrorist attack? Diagnosis, initial care, management and follow up care. A Respiratory therapist will be in a situation to prove just how valuable their presence is within the hospitals because they will be demonstrating the skills of their profession.

8. List three possible indicators of a chemical release.

Headaches
Blurred vision
Salivation

9. Describe the basic treatment for severe cyanide intoxication. Remove clothing, decontaminate victim and administration of sodium nitrate. Sodium nitrate oxidizes Hb's $Fe+2$ to produce methemoglobin's $Fe+3$. The result is the resumption of cytochrome activity and production of ATP.

10. What is the difference between pandemic and epidemic? A pandemic effects a wide geographic location and an exceptionally high proportion of people. An epidemic affects a large number of people in a given population or community.

Thought Questions

1. List at least three movies you have seen that featured a disaster likely to produce multiple casualties. Now, imagine that the disaster occurred in your area.

   a. What kinds of casualties are you likely to see? Contagion, outbreak & The Day after Tomorrow.

   ?

   b. How would the hospitals handle the influx of casualties? Hospitals would refer to NIMS as a standard and most importantly, they would follow their ICS and EOP. The ICS and EOP are the hospital's coordinated response to an incident and the EOP is the first step they would take in the emergency. These plans should tie in closely to the NIMS, which was put in place by government.

2. Think about your geographic area. What kinds of disasters have occurred? What disasters are most likely to occur? *When I think in terms of our area, I think we would be more likely to experience a tornado, earthquake or some type of chemical explosion because of the numerous factories in the area. I know we have previously experienced a couple of small earthquakes.*

3. How well would you say the hospitals in your area are prepared for an attack of bioterrorism? *I would like to think that they are prepared for anything, but I realize that mass amounts of supplies & equipment cost more money, so I'm not sure. I know that hospitals have strict regulations and protocols in place so would think that they are as ready as any other hospital.*

4. What steps must be taken by hospitals in the event of a pandemic? *HVAC must have an excess of 6 air exchanges per hr. & filtered, Flu shots must be administered to all staff as early in the flu cycle as practicable, an adequate supply of gowns & N95 masks must be in stock, aerosols & aerosol therapy must be reduced or eliminated. All exhalation from mechanically ventilated patients must be filtered using a HEPA filter and staff should decontaminate or shower & change clothes before going home.*

REVIEW

True or False

_F_   1. An earthquake that registers 3 on the Richter scale will cause damage to some buildings and cause people to flee.

_T_   2. An Injury Severity Score of greater than 25 is considered high.

_T_   3. A flood will produce casualties similar to those of hurricanes.

_F_   4. Low-order explosions are rarely lethal.

_T_   5. The shock wave from a primary blast travels faster through liquids and solids.

_F_   6. Smallpox was never declared eradicated.

_F_   7. Tabun is a pulmonary agent.

_T_   8. Children can shed an influenza virus before they are ill.

_F_   9. When caring for pandemic victims for whom bronchodilators are necessary, aerosols are better than MDIs.

_T_   10. Conservative fluid administration and aggressive use of diuretics have been shown to help reduce the duration of mechanical ventilation in patients with ARDS.

Multiple Choice

1. According to recommendations, the EMCC should include which of the following?

    1. IV fluid resuscitation
    2. vasopressor administration
    3. sedation and analgesia
    4. mechanical ventilation

    a. 1, 2, 4
    b. 1, 2, 3, 4

    c. 2, 3
    d. 2, 3, 4

2. Secondary blast injuries are more likely to occur from which of the following?

    a. burns
    b. toxic inhalation

    c. ballistic debris
    d. shock waves

3. Smallpox is normally transmitted by which of the following?

    a. droplet nuclei
    b. airborne

    c. contact
    d. ingestion

4. The single most important practice in infection control is which of the following?

    a. maintaining protective isolation
    b. prophylactic use of broad-spectrum antibiotics

    c. strict observance of universal precautions
    d. good hand hygiene

5. A patient presents who has been exposed to sarin. As a respiratory therapist, you should be concerned with which of the following effects?

    a. pneumonia
    b. metabolic acidosis

    c. tachycardia
    d. bronchospasm

Adult Critical Care

INTRODUCTION

The critical care environment is a challenge for any caregiver. With new technologies arriving daily, keeping up is hard. Caregivers who accept new challenges well should survive in this environment. Respiratory therapists are trained to function in the critical care environment and should flourish in the setting.

Discussion Activities and Questions

1. Describe the difference between APACHE and SOFA.

2. Describe a care plan. How is it used?

3. What is the primary purpose of metabolic monitoring?

4. Describe the effect of nutrition on weaning from mechanical ventilation.

5. What are the three types of intensive care units?

6. List at least three areas in the ICU in which respiratory therapists are the logical caregivers to become experts.

7. List at least five skills for which respiratory therapists can be cross-trained, along with RNs.

8. What is Level I evidence?

9. What is the difference between a clinical practice guideline and a therapist-driven protocol?

10. List at least two examples of shared policies.

Thought Questions

1. Do the ICUs that you have rotated through use a severity rating scale (e.g., SOFA, SAPS, etc.)? If so, which one?

2. Review at least three care plans for ICU patients (you might have to ask nursing). What do these have in common?

3. Compare ventilator flow sheets from hospitals in your area. How are they the same? How are they different?

4. Are the ICUs in your general area open or closed?

5. Think about your personal career goals and preferred work style. Would you rather be permanently assigned to an ICU, or would you prefer to rotate through different units in the hospital?

6. Consider the ICUs you have been in. Can you think of ways to reduce or contain costs?

7. In your experience, what are the types of patients who most commonly have required mechanical ventilation?

REVIEW

True or False

_____ 1. Patients can be admitted to the ICU directly from the cardiac catheterization lab.

_____ 2. Severity rating systems are well suited for determining therapist-to-patient ratios.

_____ 3. Stable ICU patients weaning from mechanical ventilation generally require more involvement by RTs.

_____ 4. The RT is probably the best clinician to determine a patient's readiness to wean from mechanical ventilation.

_____ 5. Generally, sepsis decreases metabolism.

_____ 6. Daily activities in the ICU do not have a significant effect on caloric requirements.

_____ 7. Implementation of ventilator weaning protocols have been shown to reduce time on mechanical ventilation.

_____ 8. Renal function can be affected by mechanical ventilation.

Multiple Choice

1. Which of the following are more advanced respiratory care procedures?
   1. airway care
   2. mechanical ventilation
   3. aerosol therapy
   4. end-tidal CO_2 monitoring

   a. 1, 2, 3
   b. 1, 2, 4
   c. 2, 3
   d. 2, 3, 4

2. Which of the following best describes the primary purpose of metabolic monitoring?

   a. assessment of oxygenation
   b. determination of cardiac output requirements
   c. determination of carbon dioxide production
   d. nutritional assessment

3. Which of the following will decrease the respiratory quotient?

   a. hyperventilation
   b. hypoxia
   c. ketogenesis
   d. carbohydrate oxidation

4. HR, a 60-year-old male on mechanical ventilation, recorded an RSBI of 78 after undergoing a spontaneous breathing trial for 90 minutes. What should the RT recommend at this point?

   a. place patient back on volume control
   b. place patient on SIMV
   c. extend the spontaneous breathing trial for another 90 minutes
   d. extubate

5. A 20-year-old male is being transferred to your ICU. It is reported that he has a fracture of C-2. Which of the following should you anticipate?

   a. He will require high-flow oxygen.
   b. He will require CPAP with pressure support.
   c. He will require careful monitoring.
   d. He will require full ventilator support.

Subacute and Long-Term Care

INTRODUCTION

With the advent and proliferation of subacute care, we have found that the respiratory therapist definitely has a role. Many specialty units, such as ventilator care units, require the respiratory care practitioner to be able to work independently. RTs can be successful in their facility by setting up a program that fits well with the needs of surrounding area hospitals. These programs need to accept both weaning and long-term ventilator patients.

Many managed care organizations are constantly seeking specialty ventilator units to contract with in an effort to reduce the overall health-care costs to their subscribers. Managed care organizations are also looking for facilities that are accredited by the Joint Commission as a sign of excellence. Because the field of subacute care continues to grow, there will continue to be changes in regulation and reimbursement. Finally, with the growing aging population in the United States, there has been an increasing need for long-term care (LTC). Although LTC can be provided to individuals of any age, most recipients of LTC are elderly and are cared for in the home, assisted living residences, specialty units, and nursing homes. The respiratory therapist can provide care in any of these venues and become a valuable member of the interdisciplinary team.

Discussion Activities and Questions

1. According to the American Health Care Association, subacute care is _____ treatment.

2. List at least four different medical reasons or conditions that can be treated in subacute care facilities.

3. Give two examples of special resources that might be found in a subacute facility.

4. Describe the difference between a nursing home and a skilled nursing facility.

5. What is a case manager?

6. What did the Muse Report indicate with regard to cost effectiveness?

7. List at least four bedside respiratory care modalities for basic and intermediate-level patients in subacute care facilities.

8. Describe at least two reasons why the cost of caring for a patient on mechanical ventilation is generally less than the costs in an acute care hospital.

9. A patient with a tracheostomy who receives mechanical ventilation at night is about to be discharged to home. List the equipment needed and the instructions to the caregivers.

10. What are some differences between assisted living facilities and nursing homes?

Thought Questions

1. Talk with respiratory therapists who work or have worked in subacute care. How does their experience differ from that of a hospital-based therapist?

2. As a student, have you had the experience of working with patients in the ICU who apparently could not be weaned from mechanical ventilation and just seemed to "disappear"? Determine where these patients went.

3. Investigate the acute care hospitals in your general area. Have any of them converted beds from acute care to subacute care in the past 15 years?

4. You are the day-shift respiratory therapist in a 90-bed subacute facility. CK, a 70-year-old female, is being transferred to your facility because she suffered a stroke that partially paralyzed her. She has a history of COPD. What should your initial assessment include and how would you proceed?

REVIEW

True or False

_____ 1. Postacute and subacute mean basically the same thing.

_____ 2. Subacute care is provided almost exclusively at nursing homes.

_____ 3. Respiratory therapists cannot be case managers.

_____ 4. Most patients requiring basic respiratory care in subacute care are typically cared for by RNs and LPNs.

_____ 5. Any subacute facility that accepts ventilator patients should have respiratory therapists on staff.

Multiple Choice

1. All of the following are traditionally acute care procedures that can be provided in subacute facilities except:

   a. surgery
   b. wound care

   c. AIDS care
   d. weaning from mechanical ventilation

2. According to the Social Security Act, patients must undergo a stay of how many days before they can be transferred to a subacute facility?

   a. 1
   b. 2

   c. 3
   d. 4

3. Specific procedures related to ventilatory support in the subacute setting include all of the following except:

   a. tracheostomy care
   b. endotracheal suctioning

   c. providing patient and caregiver training
   d. discharge planning

4. Typically, the admissions team at a subacute facility includes which of the following?

   1. nurse
   2. social worker
   3. case manager
   4. physical therapist

   a. 1, 4
   b. 1, 2, 3, 4

   c. 2, 3
   d. 3 only

5. A 67-year-old male has been admitted to your 10-bed subacute ventilator unit. He suffered an exacerbation of COPD that required intubation and mechanical ventilation. He failed multiple attempts at ventilator removal. He has a tracheostomy tube and is alert, oriented, and medically stable. You have him on the Pulmonetics LTV 1200 ventilator in volume control assist/control. Which of the following would be the best method of trying to wean him from the ventilator?

   a. Change to CPAP.
   b. Try a spontaneous breathing trial.

   c. Change to pressure control.
   d. Change to SIMV with pressure support.

Respiratory Home Care

INTRODUCTION

This chapter reviewed all the major components of a respiratory home care program, beginning with the discharge planning process. The different modalities and types of equipment were covered in depth. Assessment, patient education, and care planning processes were discussed. These are the foundation for the clinical services of the respiratory therapist. Last, the important issues of reimbursement, regulation, accreditation, and licensure were presented.

The respiratory therapist's role in home care has increased and changed over the last two decades.

Today, the respiratory therapist is a respected member of the home care team. The RT's role is based on technology developed for use in the home care setting. New technology, patient education, disease management, and pressure from payers to treat patients in the least expensive setting all cause the respiratory therapist's role in home care to increase. The challenges of reimbursement continue to be a burden for the providers of home care services. Overall, home care continues to be an exciting and challenging setting for the respiratory therapist.

Discussion Activities and Questions

1. According to the AARC, what is the goal of home respiratory care?

2. List five items in the selection criteria for home care based therapy.

3. You are asked to qualify a patient for home oxygen. Describe how you would go about it.

4. Explain, in simple terms, how a molecular sieve concentrator works.

5. Explain, in simple terms, how a liquid oxygen system works.

6. What are the differences among the three types of oxygen-conserving devices?

7. Describe at least three different methods of applying bronchial hygiene in the home.

8. List the criteria that a patient must meet to qualify for NPPV.

9. What three alarms are on an infant apnea monitor?

10. What is the function and purpose of the Joint Commission with regard to accrediting HME companies?

Thought Questions

1. What can you do to help the reimbursement situation for companies that provide home respiratory equipment?

2. If you were considering a career in respiratory home care, what qualifications do you believe you should possess?

3. You are a respiratory therapist working for an HME dealer. You set up CPAP units on several patients. What are some of the methods of monitoring patient compliance with these units?

4. When considering humidification for a patient on mechanical ventilation in the home, do you think a water-based humidifier or a heat and moisture exchanger would be better? Why?

5. You are asked to perform an assessment on a 70-year-old female who was recently discharged from the hospital. She has stage III COPD and has been prescribed oxygen at 2 Lpm. What parameters would you assess?

6. You are also asked to perform an environmental assessment on the residence of the patient in question 5. What would you assess?

REVIEW

True or False

_____ 1. Given the right conditions, any procedure can be delivered, performed, or administered to a patient at home.

_____ 2. According to CMS guidelines, PRN orders for oxygen are acceptable.

_____ 3. Liquid is the most commonly used method of delivering oxygen in the home.

_____ 4. An oxygen concentrator has been developed from which a patient can transfill a portable oxygen cylinder.

_____ 5. The pendant cannula is a type of oxygen-conserving device.

_____ 6. Battery-operated compressors used to power small-volume nebulizers are not available.

_____ 7. A home care company can do a sleep study in a patient's home, then set up the ordered CPAP unit.

—— 8. Negative pressure ventilation is the preferred method of treating patients who have ventilatory failure secondary to COPD.

—— 9. A technology-dependent child is from birth to 21-years-old.

—— 10. Once a home care patient stabilizes, the respiratory therapist never needs to review the patient's care plan.

—— 11. Under CMS requirements, an HME provider must make a concerted effort to collect the Medicare copayment.

Multiple Choice

1. All of the following are diagnoses that might qualify a patient for home respiratory care except:

   a. systemic arterial hypertension
   b. bronchiolitis
   c. pulmonary fibrosis
   d. lung cancer

2. MC is a 78-year-old male who is being discharged to an assisted living facility following an exacerbation of COPD. He has qualified for continuous home oxygen. Which of the following would be the best system to use?

   a. liquid with E cylinders for backup
   b. H cylinders
   c. concentrator with E cylinder backup
   d. concentrator with liquid for backup

3. Which of the following best describes demand flow devices?

   a. delivers flows of 2–4 Lpm during inspiration
   b. delivers flows of 1–5 Lpm continuously
   c. delivers flows within the first part of inspiration
   d. delivers a variable flow throughout inspiration

4. A ventilator-dependent patient is going home with a power chair. He wants the lightest-weight ventilator available. Which of the following ventilators should he use?

   a. iVent
   b. PLV-102
   c. Achieva
   d. LTV 1200

5. Accreditation surveys are normally done every 3 years. However, a survey can be conducted how soon after the last survey?

   a. 6 months
   b. 12 months
   c. 18 months
   d. 24 months

Pulmonary Rehabilitation

INTRODUCTION

Pulmonary rehabilitation is a challenging specialty that is rapidly growing. The respiratory therapist who wants to enter this field must be knowledgeable about various aspects of pulmonary rehabilitation, including definition and scope, patient evaluation and selection, required resources, program design and implementation, assessment and documentation of patient outcomes, and methods of obtaining reimbursement for care provided.

Pulmonary rehabilitation, though in existence since the 1950s, is actually in its infancy. Acceptance of this methodology of care for chronic lung patients is becoming an integral part of continuing respiratory care, especially at alternative sites of care. Stud-

ies have indicated the potential benefits of pulmonary rehab, yet much more needs to be done. Practitioners must continue to document the benefits of pulmonary rehabilitation in order to establish a more effective reimbursement mechanism. The CMS-funded NETT study should provide interesting results regarding the validity of pulmonary rehabilitation and reimbursement for it. In the meantime, practitioners need to work closely with their colleagues to design and implement more patient-specific and effective rehabilitation programs. With ever-increasing recognition, pulmonary rehabilitation seems to be headed on a course that will make it an essential part of long-term patient care.

Discussion Activities and Questions

1. List some of the principal differences between cardiac and pulmonary rehab programs.

2. Describe the vicious cycle of chronic pulmonary impairment.

3. Describe the consequences of abnormal pulmonary mechanics.

4. What is meant by "anaerobic threshold"?

5. List six components of the CPX test.

6. List at least four assessment parameters that should be included in a prerehabilitation patient workup.

7. What are the major differences between open-format and closed-format pulmonary rehab programs?

8. List at least five supply items you would need to stock in your outpatient pulmonary rehab program. Why do you need these supplies?

9. How is diaphragmatic breathing with pursed lips beneficial to patients with COPD?

10. List four topics you would include in the education portion of the pulmonary rehab program. Why are these important?

Thought Questions

1. Find and describe the components of the Borg dyspnea scale. Do you think this scale could also be applied to hospitalized patients?

2. You are asked to start an outpatient pulmonary rehabilitation program at your local hospital. The administrator asks what you would need to make the program successful.

   a. What do you ask for?

   b. How will you get reimbursement?

3. You are a respiratory department manager and are responsible for selecting a therapist to staff your pulmonary rehab program. What qualities and qualifications should you look for in making your selection?

4. As a staff respiratory therapist in a medium-size hospital with a pulmonary rehab program, what are some things you could do to encourage patients in the program upon discharge (assuming they meet the inclusion criteria)?

REVIEW

True or False

—— 1. Pulmonary rehab and cardiac rehab share the same goals.

—— 2. Ventilator-dependent patients are generally excluded from pulmonary rehab programs.

—— 3. The ACCP drafted the first definition of pulmonary rehab in 1942.

—— 4. COPD is ranked as the second leading cause of permanent disability in males over the age of 40.

—— 5. Hypoxemia during exercise is common in COPD patients.

—— 6. Usually, METs will be increased in patients with cardiovascular disease.

—— 7. Patients with obstructive sleep apnea might benefit from pulmonary rehab.

—— 8. It is not important for patients to enroll in and complete a nicotine intervention program prior to beginning the rehab program.

—— 9. Breathing retraining exercises can be taught at the bedside to inpatients.

—— 10. Practitioners should actively assist their patients when completing postrehab surveys.

Multiple Choice

1. Definitions of pulmonary rehabilitation generally include all of the following concepts and components except:

   a. goal of reversing the disease
   b. medical direction and involvement
   c. multidisciplinary approach
   d. multiple forms of treatment

2. Which of the following is one of the key parameters established by the cardiopulmonary exercise test?

   a. airways resistance
   b. maximal left ventricular stroke volume
   c. oxygen consumption during exercise
   d. target heart rate

3. BG is a 71-year-old female with stage III COPD. She lives with her son on the family farm. Her doctor believes she might benefit from some type of pulmonary rehab. Because of her circumstances, which of the following would probably be the most appropriate for her?

   a. open format
   b. closed format
   c. group sessions
   d. individual sessions

4. A standard in many pulmonary rehab programs is which of the following?

   a. 12-minute walk
   b. 1-mile walk
   c. 1 mile on the stationary bicycle
   d. 10-minute swim

5. The *Medicare/Medicaid Coverage Manual* indicates that respiratory therapy can entail pulmonary rehab techniques that include which of the following?

   a. appropriate aerosol therapy
   b. chest physiotherapy
   c. positive pressure breathing
   d. breathing retraining

CHAPTER 37

Patient Transport in Respiratory Care

INTRODUCTION

When transporting critically ill patients, safety is paramount. However, many patients are transported within or between health-care facilities because they are critically ill and need special services or procedures. The additional stress that may be imposed on such patients can be clinically challenging. However, through proper planning and execution and follow-up, these risks can be minimized. By following the procedures outlined in this chapter, including maintaining a state of readiness, properly prescreening patients, selecting the most appropriate means of transportation, and ensuring that the proper personnel and equipment are in place, potential complications can be avoided and patient safety can be maximized during transporting.

Discussion Activities and Questions

1. What five steps are required for successful patient transport?

2. Describe at least two factors that can increase patient stress during a transport.

3. List at least two reasons why a critically ill patient might be transported within the hospital.

4. A 70-year-old female presents to a small community hospital experiencing an exacerbation of congestive heart failure. The decision is made to transport her to the area tertiary care center. As the transport team arrives, she develops ventricular tachycardia. Should the patient be transported at this time? Why or why not?

5. During the transport of a patient who is receiving full ventilatory support, the ventilator malfunctions. How would you recognize this and what would you do first?

Thought Questions

1. Have you observed or participated in an intrahospital transport? If so, describe the patient, the purpose, and the circumstances. If not, ask your instructor or an experienced respiratory therapist.

2. You are asked to assist in the transport of an adult patient to MRI. The patient has, among other things, severe pneumonia and is being mechanically ventilated on the following settings:

Volume control

Rate	12 bpm
Tidal volume	500 mL
F_IO_2	.50
Flow	50 Lpm, decelerating
PEEP	5 cmH$_2$O

It is estimated that the transport will take about 10 minutes. Describe the factors you need to consider in the planning and execution of the transport.

REVIEW

True or False

_____ 1. A respiratory therapist should accompany all patients being transported in the hospital.

_____ 2. When planning a transport, infection control should be considered.

_____ 3. During a transport, the patient is generally not affected by additional stress.

_____ 4. The safe arrival of the mechanically ventilated patient at his or her destination is the indicator of a favorable outcome.

_____ 5. During a transport, universal precautions need not be observed.

_____ 6. Pulse oximetry readings are affected by altitude.

_____ 7. Volume-limited ventilators that use turbines will tend to deliver less than set volumes at altitude.

Multiple Choice

1. A 45-year-old male is being transported to a regional cardiac catheterization lab because he has experienced severe chest pain. Which of the following credentials should each of the transport team members possess?

   a. NRP
   b. BLS
   c. PALS
   d. ACLS

2. Which of the following has been successful in reducing stress when transporting ill neonates?

   a. mechanical ventilation
   b. specially designed isolette
   c. induced hypothermia
   d. sedation

3. Which of the following is a potential hazard of hyperventilation during transport?

   a. metabolic acidosis
   b. airway trauma
   c. hypoxemia
   d. respiratory alkalosis

4. A patient who has been successfully resuscitated following a cardiac arrest is to be transported to a regional medical center 50 miles away. Which of the following is the best mode of transport, assuming the weather is transport neutral?

   a. helicopter
   b. private ambulance
   c. critical care ambulance
   d. fixed-wing aircraft

5. You are transporting a mechanically ventilated patient. The F_IO_2 at sea level is .50. Which of the following is the equivalent F_IO_2 when cruising at an altitude of 5000 feet?

   a. .48
   b. .55
   c. .60
   d. .73

Miscellaneous Applications

Protecting the Patient and the Health-Care Provider

INTRODUCTION

Many of the microorganisms in the health-care setting do not cause respiratory illness. However, respiratory therapists encounter them regularly in patients with traditional and drug-resistant infections who also have respiratory disease that requires treatment, or in critically ill patients who need mechanical ventilatory support for respiratory failure. Thus, a thorough understanding of the chain of infection and Standard Precautions is an essential element of every RT's practice. In modern practice, the RT does not focus on respiratory disease alone. Respiratory therapists often care for patients with multisystem involvement, which, more often than not, includes infectious disease. Because critically ill patients are compromised hosts and are likely to undergo invasive procedures, such as endotracheal intubation, their risk of developing infections is extremely high.

Each RT must make a commitment to follow all infection control procedures and to keep up-to-date as recommendations change. Only a multidisciplinary effort by all members of the health-care team can keep infectious diseases under control and protect patients and health-care workers.

Discussion Activities and Questions

1. Briefly describe the chain of infection.

2. What does it mean to say that a microorganism is highly pathogenic?

3. What is the difference between a case and a carrier?

4. In microbiology, what is a "vector"?

5. List at least five factors that might make a patient more susceptible to infection.

6. Discuss the importance of hand hygiene.

7. Explain the precautions used when a patient is at risk for transmitting an airborne pathogen (e.g., TB).

8. Describe a set of symptoms or clinical presentation that would require empiric isolation precautions.

9. List the two most common multiple-drug-resistant microorganisms.

10. Briefly explain the mechanism by which a microorganism can become drug resistant.

Thought Questions

1. Respiratory departments commonly have large pieces of equipment that come in contact with patients (e.g., ventilators). Describe how this equipment is typically disinfected.

2. When you go to the hospital for clinical experience, you may see patients in isolation.

   a. What are some reasons why patients may be in isolation?

   b. What are some typical precautions caregivers are supposed to take when encountering patients in isolation?

3. Find the policy and procedure for hand hygiene in at least two of the hospitals in your local area. Do these match published standards?

4. Consider the hospitals through which you have rotated.

   a. What policies and procedures do they have in place to minimize the risk of accidental needlestick injuries?

   b. What have these hospitals done to accommodate caregivers who have latex allergies?

c. What precautions are they taking to minimize the incidence of nosocomial infection, especially ventilator-associated pneumonia, in the intensive care unit?

REVIEW

True or False

_T_ 1. An infectious agent is also called a pathogen.

_T_ 2. Hand hygiene can help stop disease transmission.

_F_ 3. Blood is a common portal for a carrier.

_F_ 4. When treating a patient who has TB, the caregiver should wear a standard surgical mask.

_T_ 5. Resident flora is also referred to as endogenous flora.

_F_ 6. As a general rule, hand hygiene is preferred over hand sanitizers.

_F_ 7. To perform closed suctioning on a ventilator patient, you should wear sterile gloves.

_T_ 8. There is no evidence that routine use of gowns to enter specific patient areas has any benefit.

_F_ 9. A health-care worker who wears eyeglasses does not need to wear goggles or a face shield.

_F_ 10. A health-care worker has a very good chance of contracting HIV from an accidental needlestick.

_T_ 11. Infectious organisms can be cultured from persons who are not ill.

Multiple Choice

1. Which of the following is not a common fomite?

   a. bedpan
   b. bed rails
   c. nebulizers
   d. metered-dose inhalers

2. Which of the following is an example of a microorganism that is commonly transmitted via direct contact?

   a. mycobacterium
   b. aspergillus
   c. legionella
   d. hepatitis

3. Which of the following is a simple and effective method of eliminating transient flora?

   a. antibiotic administration
   b. hand hygiene
   c. vigorous antisepsis
   d. oral care

4. You are assisting with the care of a patient who is receiving ventilatory support. While holding the patient over on his side so the nurse can clean the perineal area, you observe the ventilator become disconnected from the patient's tracheostomy tube. What should you do first?

   a. Immediately reconnect the ventilator.
   b. Call for help.
   c. Change your gloves.
   d. Silence the ventilator alarm.

5. You are about to work with a patient who has VRE. Which of the following should you do?

   a. Wear a face shield.
   b. Wear a respirator mask.
   c. Observe contact precautions.
   d. Wear a full isolation suit.

Health Promotion

INTRODUCTION

This chapter on health promotion provided an overview of the general concepts and principles associated with health promotion. It presented the various models of health, the dimensions of health, the underlying philosophy of health promotion, and the major role played by the individual and by society. It also presented a brief historical account of the factors that have affected health over the past century. This chapter identified and discussed the leading causes of death, but more importantly it identified and discussed the behaviors responsible for these leading killers. It identified the determining factors that render people ill or healthy and stressed the critical importance of lifestyle. It also presented a health continuum that was expanded and enhanced to depict both a traditional perspective as well as a health-promoting perspective. Compelling evidence was offered to support the incorporation of health promotion and disease prevention principles and practices into today's health-care delivery system.

Clearly, there is much to be gained by engaging in healthy lifestyle behaviors. Health maintenance organizations and managed care groups have affirmed the value of such practices and have endorsed the principles in their mission statements. Employers and insurers have identified the economic rewards of such practices. The federal government has vigorously embarked on four separate initiatives targeting Healthy People as a major goal of the future. It is equally obvious that respiratory therapists possess the clinical expertise to participate in this new and evolving component of health care. They are pivotally positioned every day at the bedside to provide the knowledge and skills requisite for respiratory health.

Respiratory therapists are clearly capable of engaging in community and organizational health promotion programming. Their stature, expertise, and knowledge in the art and science of cardiopulmonary care enable them to be major players in this movement. Health promotion is simply good medicine and certainly has a complementary role in the health-care system of the future. It will certainly continue to evolve, and respiratory therapists should welcome the opportunity to assume the role of health educator and to share their knowledge, skills, and abilities with the respiratory-impaired patient whom they serve.

Discussion Activities and Questions

1. How did the World Health Organization define "health" in 1947?

   "a state of complete physical, mental and social well-being t not merely the absence of disease or infirmity."

2. In some populations, lives often extend beyond the average. What are some factors that appear to account for this?

Genetics, diet, lifestyle and ones view of life.

3. Compare and contrast the definitions of mortality and morbidity. How have the figures for these changed over the past century?

Morbidity is the ratio of persons diseased to those who are well in a given community. Mortality is the number of deaths per unit of population in a specific region, age range or other group.

4. How has wellness been expressed?

"An approach to personal health that emphasizes individual responsibility for well being through the practice of health promoting lifestyle behavior."

5. What are some things older people can do to stimulate the intellectual dimension of wellness?

Community activities with other people of different backgrounds and cultures, library, exercise. etc...

6. List at least two examples of cultural norms or practices that do not encourage good health.

All you can eat buffets and dessert after dinner.

7. List at least four causes of preventable death in the United States. What can be done to minimize these?

Lung cancer, diabetes, liver disease, COPD

8. What are the four elements that studies have identified as contributing to death and sickness?

Environmental hazards
Unhealthy lifestyles
Inadequacies in health-care
Human biological factors

9. Compare the health continuum with the illness and wellness continuums.

10. How does Healthy People 2010 differ from Healthy People 2000?

Thought Questions

1. Think about patients with medical conditions (e.g., pneumonia) whom you have seen in the hospital.

    a. How do they appear relative to their chronological age?

    older and unhealthy

    b. Do they have any common traits (e.g., lifestyle, family history, age, etc.)?

    Smoking, cancers, heart disease or other things that may be in their genetic history

2. What do you believe you can do as a respiratory therapist to:

   a. live a healthier lifestyle?

   Promote healthy living to others, eat well, sleep well and make good life choices.

   b. promote wellness both to your peers and to the public?

   Communicate with people; both friends and the public about what you know and what you have seen.

3. Compare and contrast the three models of health. Which one do you believe has the most relevance to modern medicine? Why?

   I believe that the era of life style would be the most relevant in modern medicine because so many ailments are self inflicted or stem from one's life style choices.

4. What would you say is your primary locus of control? Regarding patients you have seen, what is their principal locus of control?

   My personal locus of control is myself; how I carry myself, how I live, how I learn, how I raise my family, and all of the choices I make for my family & myself.

5. Do you believe that the medical establishment should assume responsibility for promoting health lifestyles and preventing disease?

   Yes, I believe that any healthy promotions made by any establishment is positive. Especially in a hospital because the hospital & its staff are responsible for giving quality care. I believe this would include promoting healthy living in & out of the hosp.

6. A patient with early-stage COPD expresses a strong desire to quit smoking. Using the wellness model, what are some ways you can help?

- Eliminating the antecedent
- anticipating + preparing for the antecedent
- Substituting behaviors
- Breaking or scrambling the behavior chain
- a reward system
- a support system

REVIEW

True or False

_F_ 1. The best definition of health is the absence of disease.

_T_ 2. Average life span is the age at which half the members of a population have died.

_F_ 3. Our lifestyle behaviors are formed largely by chance.

_T_ 4. In the medical model, sole reliance is on biological processes.

_T_ 5. People who rely heavily on the health-care system to fix health problems created by lifestyle choices have an external locus of control.

_F_ 6. One's peer group exerts little pressure over one's choice of behaviors.

_T_ 7. Nearly half of all deaths that occur in the United States are largely preventable.

_F_ 8. The R in SMART refers to reward.

_F_ 9. There are nine phases in the PRECEDE model.

_T_ 10. The respiratory therapist is the foremost nonphysician expert in the bedside assessment and management of the respiratory-impaired patient.

Multiple Choice

1. According to the Georgia Centenarian Study, all of the following are common characteristics of centenarians except:

   a. access to medical care
   b. optimism
   c. flexibility
   d. commitment

2. As a health-care professional, you interact with your patients with warmth, compassion, and sensitivity. You are working in which dimension of wellness?

   a. spiritual
   b. occupational
   c. social
   d. emotional

3. One of the principal themes of wellness and health promotion is which of the following?

    a. reliance on the medical community
    b. belief in spiritual support systems
    c. acceptance of individual responsibility
    d. belief in the primacy of the prevailing social group

4. According to the Framingham Heart Study, which of the following is the most significant determinant of health status?

    a. heredity
    b. environment

    c. health-care organization
    d. lifestyle

5. The main cause of coronary artery disease is which of the following?

    a. persistent hypertension
    b. poor diet

    c. left ventricular hypertrophy
    d. smoking

Fundamentals of Patient Education

INTRODUCTION

When properly developed and delivered, patient education is a valuable tool that may reduce a patient's length of hospitalization and number of hospital stays, improve the quality of life, and increase the knowledge level of the patient and the respiratory therapist. Although the process may be complex, respiratory therapists should involve themselves in assessing patient needs, developing educational materials, providing support to patients, and assessing the success of intervention. Falvo summarizes patient education as being a patient right as well as a professional responsibility.[1] Educational materials developed with patient interest at heart and with the ideology of changing behaviors can deliver results in improvement in overall health care.

Discussion Activities and Questions

1. State the phrase you should remember when starting any educational endeavor. Do you believe this applies to you as a student? *The learner learns what the learner wants to learn when the learner wants to learn it.*

2. Define "goal." *Goal is a general statement of purpose & it is usually a simple item that may be measured to determine the success of a plan.*

3. What is an informal way for educators to measure outcomes?

Educator can ask questions that address the expectations for patient after the learning process is complete.

4. Describe communication in patient education. A series of behaviors that are specifically verbal & nonverbal to that stimulate inquiry between two or more persons.

5. Give an example of reflective questioning.

6. State one of Malcom Knowles's principles of adult education.

Adults use real life scenarios and situations to learn.

7. List the five stages of learning.

Precontemplative, contemplative, action maintenance & termination

8. How would you measure or determine patient compliance?

Asking the patient questions or just having conversation w/ them.

9. **Which AARC Clinical Practice Guidelines provide direction to the RT who is assigned the role of patient educator?**

   "Training the health care professional for the Role of patient and caregiver educator."

10. **List two topics that would be good to present to the community.**

    Long term affects of smoking
    asthma and allergies

11. **List two potential problems with using prepared educational materials.**

    The material may be in medical terms rather than laymans terms. and whatever the material contains may not be exactly what is needed.

Thought Questions

1. Review Table 40-1. Which learning do you believe best suits you as a student?

   I believe I have characteristics of each type of learner in different situations, but I am a hands on learner & learn best when I am directly involved.

2. You are assigned the task of teaching a recently diagnosed 7-year-old asthmatic how to use a metered-dose inhaler. What resources do you need? How much time do you think you will need? How would you approach the task?

3. You are asked to help instruct a patient who has recently been diagnosed with obstructive sleep apnea. Write two goals for this patient.

4. You are designing an educational program for a 22-year-old asthmatic. One of your goals is: The program will instruct the patient in the proper use of a metered-dose inhaler. Write two objectives for that goal and indicate how they will be measured.

5. Collect a sample of patient education material from hospitals in your area. Considering points to evalute, do you believe the material is ideal for patients? Why or why not?

6. You are asked to provide inservice education to the nursing staff on the general medical-surgical floors at your hospital. What are some topics you might present, and how would you proceed?

REVIEW

True or False

_T_ 1. The greatest value of modality-based learning is in teaching basic skills.

_F_ 2. When teaching preschool children, you should be emphatic and have a nonjudgmental attitude.

_F_ 3. When teaching toddlers, you should use analogies.

_T_ 4. Most clinicians are goal and objective oriented.

T 5. A goal should relate to a single end result.

F 6. An educational objective can be vague in stating what is expected of the learner.

F 7. "How do you breathe during the day?" is an example of an objective question.

F 8. Nonverbal eye contact and space constraints do not vary by culture.

T 9. Self-critique is important in improving your teaching.

T 10. With regard to patient education material, if the information is not copyrighted, you can adapt the content to fit your needs.

Multiple Choice

1. For education to be complete, which of the following must occur for the learner?

   a. must pass a written test
   b. must exhibit a change in behavior, skill, or attitude
   c. must write a summary of what has been learned
   d. must be able to teach others

2. Which of the following are observable characteristics indicative of modality strength?

   1. memory
   2. learning style
   3. general appearance
   4. state of health

   a. 1, 2, 3
   b. 1, 2, 4

   c. 1, 4
   d. 2, 3, 4

3. Which of the following is an example of an action verb that might be found in an objective?

   a. understand
   b. think

   c. know
   d. demonstrate

4. You are seeing BC, a 55-year-old male, for exacerbation of COPD. He asks you how to get more information about his disease and its management. The patient is demonstrating which of the following stages of learning?

   a. precontemplative
   b. contemplative

   c. action
   d. termination

5. You have been assigned to teach a patient who has COPD how to manage his disease. As you begin the instruction, the patient denies that he has COPD. What is your best strategy at this point?

   a. Continue the instruction.
   b. Stop and document the patient's statement.
   c. Gently and gradually confront the patient with reality.
   d. Give the patient written information about COPD.

REFERENCES

1. Falvo DR. *Effective Patient Education: A Guide to Increased Compliance.* 3rd ed. Sudbury, MA: Jones & Bartlett Publishers; 2004.

Management of Respiratory Care Services

INTRODUCTION

Managers must follow continuous quality improvement tenets to improve their work sites' effectiveness; however, managers or leaders must assume that continuous growth in their personal knowledge is an inherent responsibility of the professionals they lead. Individuals who hold leadership positions have described the growth of the respiratory care profession in Chapter 1 as directly dependent on activity levels in the profession. *Management* by definition is the concept of getting things done through others. The ability of respiratory therapists to perform management functions effectively may be learned and practiced during their career. Leadership, on the other hand, is the innate ability to convey a vision to others of how they should act or perform. Leadership is not so easily learned. This chapter contains information on management philosophy, management science, leadership characteristics, and operational methods for the day-to-day guidance of respiratory care professionals in their respective work sites. The concepts of leadership defy easy description or definition, although most people would say that they know a good leader when they see one.

A simple characteristic of accomplished leaders is that they provide consistent ethical and moral guidance to their charges, even when there are easier ways to accomplish a task. Effective communications abilities, both written and verbal, characterize managers and leaders that moreover move their areas of responsibility to a higher level of effectiveness.

Discussion Activities and Questions

1. What is the role of the medical director in respiratory care?

2. What is the difference between a centralized and a decentralized respiratory care department?

3. Define service line and give examples specific to respiratory care.

4. List some examples of supplies that would be included in the operational budget of the typical respiratory care department.

5. What is the advantage to belonging to a purchasing group?

6. List and describe two common methods employed by HMOs to control health-care expenditures.

7. Apart from pay, list at least two other factors to examine when considering employment options.

8. What is the primary purpose of employee discipline?

9. What is the advantage of a customized clinical information system?

Thought Questions

1. What do the respiratory care departments in your area do to track or enhance quality improvement? In your experience, do you believe that these efforts are effective?

2. Examine the structure of the respiratory care departments in your area. Are they centralized, quasi-decentralized, or decentralized?

3. Look at the respiratory care departments in your area that have the designation "cardiopulmonary."

   a. How many are there?

   b. What skills do the therapists possess that are peripheral to the basic skill set of most RTs?

4. How are work assignments typically given in the respiratory care departments in your area?

5. How do the departments in your area track and document employee competence?

6. How do the departments in your area track productivity? Think of some ways to increase productivity.

7. Do you believe that there should be a pay difference between RRTs who have an associate's degree and RRTs who have a bachelor's degree? Why or why not?

8. What do you believe is the most important motivator for employees?

REVIEW

True or False

_T_ 1. Clinical time standards are usually denoted by staffing plans that are tied directly to the number of timed work units.

_T_ 2. "Interdisciplinary teams" is the use of professional and nonprofessional stakeholders to make an impact on systems and practice.

_F_ 3. Membership in the AARC does not really benefit the profession as a whole.

_F_ 4. New AARC members initially have nothing to contribute to the profession.

_F_ 5. The bulk of hospitals nationwide are found in the university setting.

_T_ 6. A major use of interdisciplinary teams is the planning of controversial change processes.

_F_ 7. Equipment and equipment maintenance are the most significant portion of the typical respiratory care budget.

_F_ 8. According to studies, pay is at the top of the list of the most important employee issues.

_F_ 9. Results of a performance appraisal should be a surprise to the employee.

_T_ 10. The medical director is directly responsible for the quality practice of the department.

Multiple Choice

1. The principal role of TQM is which of the following?
   a. promote performance improvement activities
   b. set standards for quantity of work performed
   c. track compliance with accreditation standards
   d. provide a resource for setting reimbursement levels

2. The respiratory therapy manager is often given which of the following titles?
   a. chief administrator
   b. department coordinator
   c. clinical manager
   d. technical director

3. Which of the following is an example of wasted time during a shift that decreases planned productivity?
   a. unexpected emergencies
   b. travel time to and from work areas
   c. handwashing
   d. patient-related conversations with other caregivers

4. Assuming a rebate of 3% on purchases from a certain manufacturer, and assuming that the rebate can be used for additional purchases, how much more will the hospital be able to purchase if it spends $35,433?
   a. $943.37
   b. $1010.26
   c. $1062.99
   d. $1175.32

5. Current usage trends in respiratory care departments suggest that which of the following communication devices is best for point-of-care documentation and information sharing?
   a. handheld computer
   b. desktop computer
   c. cell phone
   d. Vocera

CHAPTER 1

Discussion Activities and Questions

1. Think about who you would consider a professional (either in health care or some other field). What makes these people professionals, in your view? Use the statements in the text as a guide.

2. Some obvious examples are nurses and physicians. You might also consider physical and occupational therapy, among many others.

3. Make a short list of the factors that drew you to being a respiratory therapist.

4. Use the history section in the core-text chapter, starting with Huang Ti and Hippocrates and moving up to the present.

5. Again, use the appropriate section in the core text to guide you, perhaps starting with the innovations of Alvin Barach.

6. *Scope of practice* refers to specific parameters placed on the practice of your profession. It is usually defined by law. It would be a good idea to look at the law that governs the practice of respiratory care in your particular state.

7. Advanced cardiac life support, pediatric advanced life support, and so on are defined by the American Heart Association. The National Board for Respiratory Care also has advanced credentials. You should also consider credentials in asthma education and sleep.

Thought Questions

1. This is a tough question to answer, mainly because this has been the history of medicine. Should we become more oriented toward wellness? If so, how do we accomplish this shift?

2. Medicare is basically insurance for the elderly (people over the age of 65); Medicaid is assistance for those who cannot afford health care.

3. Much of this shift happened in the early 1980s; it changed the dynamic of respiratory care.

4. This is another tough question. Managed care is becoming more and more a reality and provides a good opportunity for our profession.

REVIEW

True or False

1. True

2. True

3. False

Multiple Choice

1. d
2. b
3. a
4. d
5. a
6. c
7. b

CHAPTER 2

Discussion Activities and Questions

1. The answer to this question should be clear from the discussion in the core text. The main principle to extract is that legal requirements are enacted by the state and carry the force of law.

2. See Table 2-1 in the core text.

3. See Table 2-1 in the core text.

4. A *tort* is a legally defined wrong committed upon a person or property, independent of contract, that renders the individual who commits it liable for damages in a civil action. Torts are the violation of some private duty by which damages accrue to the individual and for which the courts will provide a remedy in the form of an action for damages. Think in terms of either assault (forcing a patient to accept an unwanted treatment) or negligence resulting in harm.

5. *Slander* is saying something untrue that might damage another's reputation. In health care, this could involve spreading or repeating rumors that call into question the competence of another caregiver.

6. Misappropriation, intrusion, public disclosure, presenting someone in a false light to the public (see core text for details).

7. *Double effect* is when the practitioner is faced with an ambiguous situation in which there are multiple effects from an action. One effect might be positive whereas the other might be negative. An example is doing cardiac compressions on an elderly patient who has osteoporosis.

8. Think about different religious beliefs and practices. A well-known example is the refusal of any Jehovah's Witness to accept blood transfusions. You need to consider and accommodate many different religious beliefs in your daily practice.

9. One definition is a rule of action to which people obligate themselves to conform.

10. You can find this on the AARC website (www.aarc.org). Although not legally binding, it does provide a guide for ethical practice.

Thought Questions

1. You need to check with your instructors and the policies of the education program.

2. a. To force the patient might be considered assault. The RT needs to seek help if he cannot convince the patient.

   b. Again, this might be considered assault, especially if the patient is judged to be rational at the time of the treatment refusal.

3. Any such disclosure would be a breach of confidentiality.

4. This is a question of ethics more than legalities. You must search your own conscience for the answer to what *you* would do.

5. This is a clear breach of medical ethics.

6. This is a very difficult question and situation. The RT should refer the question to the attending physician.

REVIEW

True or False

1. False
2. True
3. True
4. True
5. True
6. False
7. False
8. True

Multiple Choice

1. b
2. a
3. a
4. c
5. b
6. d
7. d
8. d
9. d
10. d

CHAPTER 3

Discussion Activities and Questions

1. *Theories* are statements that are believed to be true but that are still being tested or are doubted in some scientific circles. *Principles* are statements of perceived truths about defined situations.

2. To minimize confusion and to provide a clue as to the outcome of the mathematical formulas.

3. The *law of inertia,* or Newton's first law of motion, states that "a body at rest tends to stay at rest and a body in uniform motion tends to stay in motion unless acted upon by an outside force."

4. If you try this experiment (and do not cheat by stretching the balloon first!), you should find that the balloon is at first difficult to inflate, then gets easier, then gets difficult as it approaches its maximum capacity. This is an application of LaPlace's law. If you were to graph this, you would find that the graph resembled the compliance curve of the lung.

5. Mass is a clearly defined property of matter. Weight is mass subject to the effects of gravity.

6. Think of different types of ventilators; also, some ultrasonic nebulizers and high-flow nasal cannulas (among many other examples).

7. Should the hospital allow the patient to bring in his or her own CPAP machine, or should the hospital provide the equipment? This is controversial at present and revolves around principles of electricity, as well as hygiene.

8. Mucus must have some viscosity in order to move along the mucociliary escalator (water is very difficult to remove). However, when it gets too viscous, it tends to adhere to the airways. Clearly, one of the RT's jobs is to facilitate secretion removal.

9. Theoretically, yes, because the length of the tracheostomy tube is less than that of the endotracheal tube. However, the effect is negligible and has not been demonstrated in studies.

10. Even though the diameter of each individual bronchiole is less, the overall cross-sectional area is much greater; therefore, the resistance is lower.

11. The Venturi principle includes entrainment of surrounding fluid (generally air).

12. Normal ventilation operates using Boyle's law (i.e., when the volume of the thoracic cavity increases through the descent of the diaphragm, the pressure in the thoracic cavity decreases with respect to the atmosphere).

13. This is an application of Gay-Lussac's law (pressure is directly proportional to temperature if the volume remains the same).

14. Because the atmospheric pressure decreases as the elevation decreases, the PO_2 of the atmosphere also decreases proportionally.

15. Without surfactant, the effects of surface tension would be to collapse the alveoli. With collapsed alveoli, LaPlace's law predicts that it would take a greater distending pressure to reinflate the alveolus.

REVIEW

True or False

1. True
2. False
3. False
4. True
5. False
6. False
7. True
8. False
9. True
10. False

Multiple Choice

1. d
2. b
3. c
4. a
5. d
6. b
7. d
8. b
9. a
10. a

Lab Activities

1. This is a good and easy experiment to try. The movement of the balloon resembles that of an alveolus (think elastic recoil).

2. This is a very easy experiment to try. (This author will not bias your experiment by giving you the answer in advance.)

3. Write out Poiseuille's law, then try the experiment. It is amazing how mathematical models really can predict observable behavior.

CHAPTER 4

Discussion Activities and Questions

1. See Table 4-1 in the core text.

2. Use Table 4-1 and Figure 4-2 from the core text.

3. Carbohydrates, lipids, proteins, and nucleic acids.

4. A substance that has a molecular structure built up chiefly or completely from a large number of similar units bonded together (e.g., starch and glycogen).

5. Proteins have many functions. See the core text for examples.

6. The tendency of acids to dissociate or ionize into H_3O^+ is expressed as the *dissociation constant (k)*.

7. H_2CO_3 (carbonic acid).

8. CO_2 is carried in the blood in six different ways. The majority of CO_2 is carried as HCO_3 in the plasma.

9. Three ways in the plasma and three ways in the red blood cell (attached, dissociated, and as HCO_3).

10. pK (6.1) + log (HCO$_3$/PCO$_2$ × 0.03)

11. Facilitates the creation and dissociation of carbonic acid.

12. Deoxygenation of the blood increases its ability to carry carbon dioxide; this property is the Haldane effect. Conversely, oxygenated blood has a reduced capacity for carbon dioxide.

13. Any condition that causes the retention of carbon dioxide (usually secondary to ventilatory failure).

14. The kidney works by retaining HCO$_3$ in the loop of Henle.

15. Standard normals: (a) 7.35–7.45, (b) 80–100 mm Hg, (c) 35–45 mm Hg, (d) 22–26 mEq

16. There are more than three. However, the principal causes are lactic acidosis, ketoacidosis, and renal failure. Calculating the ion gap will help to discriminate among possible causes.

REVIEW

True or False

1. True	4. True	7. True	10. True
2. False	5. False	8. False	11. True
3. False	6. False	9. False	12. True

Multiple Choice

1. c	4. d	7. c	10. b
2. d	5. b	8. b	
3. a	6. d	9. d	

CHAPTER 5

Discussion Activities and Questions

1. Kingdom, phylum, class, order, family, genus, species.

2. Klebsiella, pseudomonas (among many others).

3. *Enzyme-linked immunosorbent assay* (*ELISA*) is a sensitive immunochemical technique that uses an enzyme-antibody-antigen combination placed in a test well.

4. See the core text for these six steps.

5. Antimicrobial susceptibility or sensitivity helps in determining the resistant ability of a microbe.

6. These are part of the normal flora of the body which, under certain circumstances, can become pathogenic. Examples are streptococcus and candida.

7. Resident bacteria can aid in inhibiting more harmful bacterial growth and also in certain biological processes (e.g., digestion).

8. Outer barriers (e.g., skin, mucus membranes) and cell-mediated responses (e.g., white blood cells).

9. The nose and lungs are the best examples, although other organs also have mucous membranes. Mucus serves to trap foreign particles, including pathogenic microorganisms.

10. A fever may stimulate white blood cells and raise the body temperature above the range preferred by bacteria.

11. Neutrophils (principal killer), eosinophils and basophils (active in the immune response), monocytes (late responders), and lymphocytes (moderate the immune response in different ways).

12. Depending on the injury, the body will manifest both an inflammatory and an immune response. Outward signs might be redness and swelling.

13. Many vaccines are currently available, including those for traditional childhood illnesses (e.g., measles, mumps, chickenpox). There are many others that help to eradicate illnesses that were at one time very serious (e.g., polio). Many people get vaccinated for influenza every year. Do you?

14. Any part of the body that is open to the environment in some way is certainly vulnerable to microbial invasion. Ironically, the respiratory tract (which is moist, warm, and full of mucus) provides a nurturing environment for many strains of bacteria.

15. *Disinfection* is the inhibition or destruction of pathogens; *sterilization*, or *asepsis*, is the complete absence or destruction of all microorganisms. You probably have some disinfectants (spray cleansers) around your home.

16. See Table 5-2 in the core text.

17. Basically, *virulence* refers to the ability of microorganisms to resist attempts to kill them.

18. • An incubation period with no symptoms

    • A prodromal, or preacute, phase in which the person feels unwell but has no symptoms

    • Acute illness with symptoms

    • Recovery, disability, or death

19. *Endemic* diseases are those that are constantly present in a population, usually involving only a few people. An *epidemic* occurs when a greater-than-normal number of cases of an endemic disease occur in an area at a specific time.

REVIEW

True or False

1. False	4. False	7. False	10. True
2. True	5. True	8. False	
3. False	6. False	9. True	

Multiple Choice

1. b	4. c	7. c	10. a
2. d	5. d	8. c	
3. a	6. d	9. a	

Matching

1. e	3. b	5. c
2. d	4. a	

Lab Activities

1. Do you have patient-oriented equipment (e.g., masks, cannulas, etc.) or ventilators in your lab?

2. What methods of disinfection/sterilization have you seen at various clinical sites?

3. Have you ever had an infection of any kind (e.g., pneumonia)?

4. Think about the last time you had the flu. If you have never been sick, have you lived with someone who has had the flu or pneumonia?

CHAPTER 6

Discussion Activities and Questions

1. The Valsalva maneuver is performed by attempting to forcibly exhale while keeping the mouth and nose closed. It can help to equalize the pressures in the sinuses and ears, which become unequal during environmental pressure changes.

2. a. Think about diseases like COPD or pneumonia, perhaps even cystic fibrosis.

   b. Damage could lead to retained and/or dried secretions, which could lead to pneumonia or airway blockage.

   c. Think about the various therapeutic adjuncts used to facilitate secretion removal (e.g., bronchial hygiene).

3. Smooth muscles constrict, mucus accumulates, and the airways become inflamed. The usual treatment is to give bronchodilators and anti-inflammatories.

4. Surfactant reduces the surface tension around the alveoli. Without it, the alveoli would tend to collapse.

5. Compare the sympathetic branch with the parasympathetic branch.

6. Because of the angle of the right mainstem bronchus (look at the configuration of the two mainstem bronchi at the carina).

7. One glides over the other during inspiration. If they dry out or become inflamed, inspiration becomes very painful.

8. Look at Poiseuille's law and apply it to the airway.

9. Time constant = compliance × resistance.

10. *Dead space ventilation* refers to gas that does not participate in gas exchange. The normal way to calculate anatomic dead space is 1 mL per pound ideal body weight.

11. Generally, ventilation becomes more difficult and the respiratory pattern becomes rapid and shallow.

12. What do these prefixes mean? Sometimes we use these terms interchangeably (often including hyperventilation); however, each does have a distinct meaning and should be used precisely.

13. Think about the two different circulations (pulmonary versus systemic). The left ventricle has a much harder job.

14. Lungs versus the rest of the body (the pulmonary circulation does have some unique properties).

15. Preload, afterload, and contractility.

16. The *Bohr effect* occurs when an increase of carbon dioxide (CO_2) in the blood results in the dissociation of oxygen (O_2) from hemoglobin.

17. The wider the gap between the two contents, the lower the cardiac output.

18. There are many potential causes of shunting. These can be either cardiac (e.g., left to right shunt) or pulmonary (e.g., pneumonia).

19. The kidney works by retaining HCO_3 in the loop of Henle.

20. Alveolar minute ventilation divided by cardiac output. What is the normal?

21. The *respiratory quotient* (*RQ*) reflects internal tissue gas exchange (internal respiration). The *respiratory exchange ratio* (*REQ*) measures external pulmonary gas exchange between the alveoli and the atmosphere per minute.

22. This is a complex process that revolves around how the diffusion of carbon dioxide into the cerebral spinal fluid decreases the pH.

23. This is a controversial process. It involves the response curve of the peripheral chemoreceptor (decreasing PaO_2).

24. See Figure 6-49 in the core text.

25. The primary method is to increase hemoglobin content. You might also increase cardiac output and minute volume.

REVIEW

True or False

1. False	7. False	13. True	19. True
2. True	8. True	14. True	20. False
3. False	9. False	15. False	21. False
4. True	10. True	16. False	22. True
5. False	11. True	17. False	
6. False	12. False	18. False	

Multiple Choice

1. a	5. b	9. c	13. a
2. a	6. c	10. b	14. a
3. b	7. d	11. d	
4. d	8. b	12. a	

Matching

1. b	4. b	7. d
2. a	5. a	8. a
3. a	6. b	9. c

Lab Activities

1. This is not as difficult as you might imagine. You might be able to do it to yourself in front of a mirror.

2. Not quite as realistic as a real person. However, you need to be familiar with upper airway anatomy.

3. The curve should resemble the compliance graph of the lung.

4. This is a very useful way to learn about time constants in relation to mechanical ventilation.

5. You will probably observe an increase in vital signs. During exercise, oxygen consumption goes up along with an increase in carbon dioxide production.

CHAPTER 7

Discussion Activities and Questions

1. Metered dose inhalers, small-volume nebulizers, large-volume nebulizers, and ultrasonic nebulizers.

2. Bronchodilator, mast cell inhibitor, corticosteroid.

3. Tremors, tachycardia, palpitations, headache, nausea.

REVIEW

Multiple Choice

1. a
2. b
3. c
4. d
5. b
6. a

Matching

1. c
2. d
3. a
4. b
5. f
6. g
7. e

Case Studies

1. Albuterol, because it is a rescue inhaler and the patient is in distress.

2. Combivent is the rescue inhaler and Flovent is the maintenance inhaler.

CHAPTER 8

Discussion Activities and Questions

1. When a healthy person is exposed, a granuloma surrounds the TB organism and contains it, without symptoms. If a person is immunocompromised, the granuloma can rupture, allowing the disease-causing organisms to spread; the patient will develop an actual infection and become symptomatic.

2. Coccidiodomycosis (southwest United States, northern Mexico), histoplasmosis (Ohio and Mississippi River valleys), blastomycosis (north central Midwest, mid-Atlantic states, upstate New York, southern Canada, southeastern United States).

3. Viral infections are rarely fatal except in people with lowered immunity; bacterial infections are more often lethal. Viruses can be transmitted by inhalation or direct upper-airway contact; bacterial pneumonia, such as community-acquired pneumonia, occurs mainly from aspiration in the lower respiratory tract (in particular the oropharynx).

Thought Question

1. It is important to educate HIV-positive patients, especially patients who also carry risk factors for TB. Literature at clinics as well as education by staff may help bring better awareness.

REVIEW

Multiple Choice

1. d	3. b	5. d	7. a
2. a	4. b	6. a	8. g

Matching

1. d	2. a	3. c	4. b

CHAPTER 9

Discussion Activities and Questions

1. Refer to Table 9-1 in the core text.

2. Acute phase (bronchospasm, secretions, mucosal edema); subacute phase (initial symptoms are treated, inflammatory pattern still present); chronic inflammation phase (inflammation that maintenance therapy attempts to control).

3. *Idiopathic, postinfection, and underlying disease:* Secondary genetic immunologic dysfunction or autoimmune abnormalities; genetic causes, such as cystic fibrosis, primary immotile cilia syndrome, and alpha-1 antitrypsin deficiency; IgG immune deficiency and immune-related dysfunction, such as allergic bronchopulmonary aspergillosis collagen vascular diseases and inflammatory bowel diseases; chronic gastric aspiration, foreign body aspiration, and endobronchial tumors; COPD and asthma.

Thought Questions

1. Short-acting beta-2 drugs would be the appropriate choice, as they will act fastest.

2. Items to look for could include social history, cigarette smoking history, and environmental exposure, among others.

REVIEW

Multiple Choice

1. c
2. a

3. d
4. g

5. f

Matching

1. b
2. e

3. c
4. a

5. d

CHAPTER 10

Discussion Activities and Questions

1. Idiopathic pulmonary fibrosis, acute interstitial pneumonia, desquamate interstitial pneumonia, non-specific interstitial pneumonia.

2. Rock mining, rock quarrying, tunneling, foundry work, manufacturing, sandblasting, stonecutting.

3. Reduced DLCO, reduced TLC, reduced FEV_1.

REVIEW

Multiple Choice

1. b
2. c

3. a
4. f

5. a
6. c

7. a
8. b

Matching

1. b
2. d

3. e
4. a

5. b

Case Study

1. Other tests might include: PFT, ABG, chest X-ray, high-resolution CT scan, bronchoalveolar lavage, diffusion study, VATS procedure for definitive diagnosis.

CHAPTER 11

Discussion Activities and Questions

1. Smoking, air pollution, certain occupations such as uranium and asbestos work, radon gas exposure, hormonal influences.

2. Dyspnea, tachypnea, fever, low SPO_2, dullness to percussion, diminished or absent breath sounds in the affected area, tracheal deviation to the affected side.

3. Respiratory distress, dyspnea, chest pain usually on affected side, low SPO_2, subcutaneous emphysema, reduced or absent breath sounds on affected side, hyper-resonance to percussion on affected side, tracheal deviation away from affected side.

REVIEW

Multiple Choice

1. b
2. b
3. b
4. d
5. a
6. f
7. c

Matching

1. b
2. f
3. d
4. c
5. e

Case Studies

1a. Spontaneous pneumothorax; the patient is a male between the ages of 20 and 40 with a history of cigarette smoking.

1b. Absence of vascular markings on the affected side, possible tracheal deviation away from affected side.

1c. Thoracentesis, chest tube placement afterward.

CHAPTER 12

Discussion Activities and Questions

1. Emphysema, chronic bronchitis, chronic asthma, kyphoscoliosis, diffuse parenchymal lung diseases, sarcoidosis, obstructive sleep apnea, obesity hypoventilation syndrome, neuromuscular diseases, pulmonary hypertension, pulmonary vasculitis.

2. Loop diuretics (furosemide), ACE inhibitors, angiotensin receptor blockers, morphine, dopamine, dobutamine, norepinephrine, nesiritide, phosphodiesterase inhibitors.

3. Sudden onset, risk factor for ARDS, poor gas exchange (refractory hypoxemia), diffuse bilateral infiltrates on X-ray, pulmonary capillary wedge pressure < 18 mm Hg.

REVIEW

Multiple Choice

1. c
2. a

3. b
4. d

5. b
6. a

Matching

1. e
2. b

3. a
4. f

5. d

Case Studies

1a. Cardiogenic pulmonary edema

1b. CPAP

CHAPTER 13

Discussion Activities and Questions

1. Verbal and nonverbal techniques that indicate comprehension.

2. Adventitious can also be considered abnormal breath sounds.

3. Auscultation can be performed when listening for bowel sounds or maneuvers such as whispering petroliloquy or egophony.

4. Intimate space is where the actual physical assessment is performed.

REVIEW

Multiple Choice

1. d
2. a

3. a
4. b

5. b
6. a

7. d
8. c

CHAPTER 14

Discussion Activities and Questions

1. "Butterfly" appearance on the film.

2. Portable is shot from front to back, regular is shot from back to front; images on portable, such as heart shadow, will look bigger.

3. Tracheal shift away from affected side, mediastinal shift away from affected side.

4. Get information not available by physical exam, identify conditions that require urgent treatment, assess patient's response to therapy, do preliminary assessment when physician is not available, assist in proper positioning of tubes.

Thought Questions

1. Wide intercostal spaces, flattened diaphragm.

2. Chest X-ray would not be beneficial; spiral CT scan would be best.

3. Yes, one view may not always provide a complete picture.

REVIEW

Multiple Choice

1. c	3. d	5. d	7. c
2. a	4. b	6. b	

Matching

1. c	3. f	5. a
2. d	4. b	

CHAPTER 15

Discussion Activities and Questions

1. Intracellular, extracellular (plasma and interstitial fluid).

2. This is water loss that cannot be measured (think sweat and mucus—remember that mucus is mostly water).

3. This is a common problem and one you should be constantly thinking about. An artificial airway bypasses the upper airway humidification mechanisms.

4. The body attempts to maintain electroneutrality. When HCO_3 leaves the red blood cell, it must be replaced by another anion (Cl^-).

5. Low levels of magnesium may result in prolonged involuntary muscle spasms (notably in airway smooth muscle).

6. Think light wavelength analysis. See the core text, and particularly Figure 15-4, for a more complete description.

7. *Biosensors* are devices that combine ion-specific electrodes, enzymatic methodology, and solid-phase technology to selectively recognize an element with a transducer.

8. • *Coulometry* is an electrochemical titration in which the titrant is electrochemically generated and the end point is detected by amperometry.

   • *Amperometry* is measurement of a current through an electrolyte solution.

9. The answer to this question should be obvious, as accurate and believable data are paramount to providing quality care.

10. *Standard deviation (Sd)* is a measure of dispersion (the spread of the data around the mean). *Coefficient of variance (CV)* is the standard deviation expressed as a percentage of the mean.

11. Trend analysis, such as in a Levey-Jennings control chart, monitors the function of a device (in this case, an electrode) over time. This helps in watching for the emergence of defects.

REVIEW

True or False

1. True	4. False	7. True	10. True
2. False	5. True	8. True	11. False
3. True	6. False	9. False	

Multiple Choice

1. b	4. d	7. b	10. d
2. c	5. a	8. a	
3. c	6. c	9. a	

Matching

1. e	3. a	5. d
2. c	4. b	

Lab Activities

1. [Answers will be specific to the area.] You might find that in some hospitals, RTs are responsible for the analysis, whereas in others, medical technologists may be responsible. Also, do any of the clinical facilities do point-of-care testing?

2. a. Levey-Jennings graph.

   b. Quality assurance.

CHAPTER 16

Discussion Activities and Questions

1. See Figure 16-1 in the core text.

2. pH = pK (6.1) + log (HCO_3/H_2CO_3)

3. Ventilation, kidney, intracellular, extracellular.

4. Allen's test checks for collateral circulation in the wrist (radial and ulnar arteries).

5. Pulse oximetry requires sufficient circulation to generate a pulse. Also, most pulse oximeters do not discriminate between different forms of dysfunctional hemoglobin.

6. Normal lab values are statistically derived by analyzing values scattered over a population.

7. Plethysmography is the basic operating principle of the pulse oximeter. *Plethysmography* is the study of changes in the shape or size of an organ.

8. The pulse oximeter does not discriminate between normal oxyhemoglobin and carboxyhemoglobin. In recent years, however, a pulse oximeter has been introduced that will discriminate.

9. The answer relates to where the sensor is located relative to the flow of exhaled gas.

10.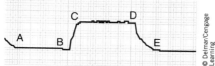

    A–B: Exhalation of dead-space gas (no CO_2)

    B–C: Exhalation from respiratory bronchioles

    C–D: Exhalation from alveoli

    D–E: End of exhalation

11. The answer is multifaceted. However, think about the relative thickness of the skin and underlying tissue.

12. See Figure 16-15 in the core text.

13. Among other things, basically the anion gap helps to discriminate between causes of metabolic acidosis.

14. Think mostly about pulse oximetry and capnography.

REVIEW

True or False

1. False
2. False
3. True
4. True

5. False
6. True
7. False
8. False

9. False
10. True
11. False
12. False

13. True

Multiple Choice

1. a
2. d
3. a

4. b
5. c
6. a

7. c
8. a
9. c

10. d
11. b
12. c

Lab Activity

1. 7.16

CHAPTER 17

Discussion Activities and Questions

1. There are many reasons to do pulmonary function testing. One is to stage lung diseases (e.g., COPD). Another is to determine response to a bronchodilator. Yet another is to determine the presence of decreased lung function. See Table 17-1 in the core text.

2. Spirometry, static lung volumes (e.g., total lung capacity, functional residual capacity), and diffusing capacity. Some labs might also include arterial blood gas testing and airway resistance. See Table 17-2 in the core text.

3. Pulmonary fibrosis, pneumoconiosis, sarcoidosis, pneumonia (among others).

4. See Figure 17-4 in the core text.

5. The curve should have a concavity as it approaches the x axis.

6. Open circuit/nitrogen washout; closed circuit/helium dilution; body plethysmography (most accurate).

7. The most likely explanation is that not enough carbon dioxide is being filtered out (remember this is a closed circuit).

8. CO is used because it is so readily picked up by the hemoglobin. It is not dangerous because it is used only in trace amounts.

9. This is the point at which normal oxygen supplies in the blood are depleted and the cells must begin to operate on anaerobic metabolism.

10. See the core text for this testing procedure.

11. To determine how reactive a patient's airways are to cholinergic stimulation.

12. There are many types of spirometers. The categories are volume-displacement and flow-sensing. Most spirometers today use some kind of pneumotachometer (flow-sensing).

REVIEW

True or False

1. True
2. False
3. False
4. True
5. True
6. False
7. False
8. False
9. True
10. False

Multiple Choice

1. c
2. c
3. d
4. a
5. a
6. b
7. d
8. c
9. a
10. c

Lab Activity

4. According to ATS guidelines, the figure shows severe obstruction with increased residual volume, no restriction, decreased diffusing capacity, and no response to bronchodilator.

CHAPTER 18

Discussion Activities and Questions

1. In bilevel therapy, inspiratory and expiratory pressure can be adjusted independent of one another. Titrating bilevel is more challenging because two separate pressure are being titrated, as opposed to one in CPAP.

2. Begins with NREM sleep progressing through stage N1 through N2 and N3, followed by an REM period in a 90-second cycle

3. In NREM sleep, minute ventilation decreases by 0.5–1.5 Lpm and respiratory rate increases. In REM sleep, the respiratory pattern varies. Upper airway resistance increases during sleep; there is a reduced functional residual capacity during sleep due to reduced respiratory muscle activity; blood pressure falls 5%–14% during NREM sleep and fluctuates during REM sleep; heart rate decreases during NREM sleep, but can vary during REM sleep and bradycardia may occur.

Thought Question

1. Restraining the patient may be beneficial; offering an alternative to a mask, such as nasal prongs, may help as well.

REVIEW

Multiple Choice

1. b   3. a   5. d   7. d
2. e   4. c   6. b   8. a

Matching

1. c   3. e   5. d
2. a   4. b

CHAPTER 19

Discussion Activities and Questions

1. Changes in SVO_2 usually precede hemodynamic changes that indicate the need to reassess the patient's status.

2. Heart rate and rhythm, quality of pulse, capillary refill, skin and mucous membrane color, skin temperature, level of consciousness, urine output, neck vein distention.

3. Ventricular fibrillation.

4. 190 bpm

REVIEW

Multiple Choice

1. b   3. d   5. b   7. c
2. a   4. d   6. a   8. d

Matching

1. c   3. a   5. b
2. d   4. e

Case Studies

1a. Complete or third-degree AV block.

1b. No relationship between the atria and the ventricles.

1c. Yes, because it can develop into asysytole.

CHAPTER 20

Discussion Activities and Questions

1. Helium is much less dense than oxygen. In diseases in which the airways are narrowed or partially blocked, helium/oxygen mixtures are more likely to move to the distal alveoli.

2. When exposed to extreme heat or cold, compressed gas will behave according to Gay-Lussac's law.

3. Liquid is much more highly compressed than gaseous oxygen. A container of liquid O_2 will hold a lot more oxygen (861 times more).

4. American Standard Safety System, Diameter Index Safety System, Pin Index Safety System.

5. See Figure 20-15 in the core text.

6. Increased heart rate, increased respiratory rate, mental confusion, headache, decreased SpO_2, decreased PaO_2.

7. The difference lies basically in how much of the gas the patient inhales with each breath actually comes from the device. In a high-flow system, the device provides 100% of what the patient is breathing.

8. A nonrebreathing system is the simplest oxygen delivery device that will provide a high percent of oxygen to the patient (usually in the 70% range).

9. See Table 20-10 in the core text.

10. See Table 20-12 in the core text.

REVIEW

True or False

1. False	4. False	7. True	10. False
2. True	5. False	8. False	11. True
3. True	6. True	9. False	

Multiple Choice

1. a	4. d	7. d
2. b	5. b	8. a
3. c	6. b	9. b

Lab Activities

1. The flowmeters are probably the same type. However, you might see that some rooms have more than one, or some rooms (particularly ICU and the ED) might have both oxygen and air flowmeters.

2. *Monitoring* means keeping track of how much oxygen is being used. Check with the department procedure manual for what to do in case of fire.

3. Large-volume nebulizers generally work on the Venturi principle. They are used primarily to provide humidified oxygen to patients who use artificial airways. If you recall air entrainment ratios, you can figure out how to increase total flow to the patient.

4. You probably do not see a lot of transcutaneous monitoring outside of a neonatal unit. Arterial blood gas analysis is still the gold standard; however, this test is invasive and expensive.

5. The pulse oximeter can measure both hemoglobin content and carboxyhemoglobin. How would these measurements be useful in a clinical setting?

6. You can also check with the AARC for additional protocols.

CHAPTER 21

Discussion Activities and Questions

1. *Relative humidity (RH)* compares the actual amount of water present in a given volume of gas (content, or AH) with the amount the gas is capable of holding at that temperature (capacity).

2. *Body humidity (BH)* is the water vapor content required to fully saturate alveolar air at normal body temperature, expressed as a percentage.

3. An *aerosol* is the suspension of particles in a gas flow. (Do not confuse this with humidity.)

4. This is an important clinical consideration. The warmer the gas and the more humid the gas flow, the more the particles will get diluted and fall out of suspension. Think about this as you administer aerosol drugs in a ventilator circuit.

5. Nonmedicated aerosol (e.g., normal saline).

6. This will, of course, depend on the device. Infection control is always an issue. You might also consider thermal burns and overhumidification.

7. A heated wire circuit decreases the rainout in the tubing.

8. See Table 21-6 in the core text.

9. Servocontrolled versus nonservocontrolled. See Figure 21-6 in the core text.

10. Slow and deep through the mouth with a breath hold.

REVIEW

True or False

1. True	4. False	7. False	10. False
2. True	5. True	8. False	
3. False	6. True	9. True	

Multiple Choice

1. a	4. b	7. b	10. a
2. c	5. d	8. b	
3. a	6. a	9. b	

Lab Activities

1. a. Mucus is produced by submucosal glands and goblet cells. Mucus is released into the sol layer, which lies below the gel layer. The cilia then propel the mucus out of the lungs.

   b. 95% water and 5% glycoproteins and lipids.

   c. Any disease that interferes with normal mucociliary function (e.g., COPD, cystic fibrosis, etc.).

2. The particles of bronchodilator must reach the smaller airways, so the particle size should be in the 2–5 micron range. You also need to consider the patient's ability in determining the appropriate nebulizer.

3. a. Specifically, look at the type(s) of nebulizers (e.g., small-volume, breath-actuated, etc.).

   b. Then look at the specifications (e.g., particle size and distribution, etc.) for each device.

   c. When you look at the specifications of different nebulizers versus the patient population, you find that some nebulizers are simply more efficient.

4. a. Specifically, do they use heated humidifiers, or HMEs, or both?

   b. If they use both, how do they decide which to use?

5. This is a good question that is difficult to answer because it has not been adequately studied. You need to consider efficacy versus efficiency.

CHAPTER 22

Discussion Activities and Questions

1. Atelectasis can be caused either by gas not being able to reach certain alveoli or the inability of the lungs and/or chest to expand (think pulmonary fibrosis, postoperative pain, etc.).

2. The alveoli are elastic bodies, which make passive exhalation possible, but also serve to make inhalation more difficult. Ventilation operates via Boyle's law.

3. The Sugarloaf Conference was the first to study the scientific foundations of IPPB. After the conference, IPPB as a mainstream therapy was called into question and slowly began to fall out of favor.

4. Pores of Kohn and canals of Lambert.

5. Slow and deep (think hyperinflation therapy).

6. See Figure 22-7 in the core text.

7. By applying positive pressure to the alveoli during exhalation, functional residual capacity will be preserved or even increased, thus potentially reversing atelectasis.

8. See procedure in the core text.

REVIEW

True or False

1. True	4. False	7. True	10. True
2. False	5. True	8. True	
3. True	6. False	9. False	

Multiple Choice

1. a
2. d
3. b
4. a
5. c

Lab Activities

1. a. Specifically, what types of devices do they have for incentive spirometry, EPAP therapy, IPPB, and so on?

   b. Is this therapy routinely administered, or just occasionally to very specific patients?

2. a. Many hospitals still set up freestanding CPAP. You will need, at least, a high-flow oxygen source, a PEEP valve, a full face mask, and tubing.

   b. This is a high-flow device, so the flow must be at least three times the patient's minute volume. Depending on the device, this may be hard to determine. F_IO_2 can be checked with an oxygen analyzer.

   c. [See answer to part b.]

CHAPTER 23

Discussion Activities and Questions

1. Mucus, sol layer, gel layer, and cilia.
2. Deep inspiration, pause at peak inspiration, compressive phase, expiratory phase.
3. There are many factors. Some include atelectasis, impaired ability to inhale, presence of artificial airway.
4. The measurement of maximum expiratory pressure (MEP) at the mouth appears to be an excellent indicator for the capacity to generate peak flow transients.
5. Clearly, you need to be sensitive to the patient's recent abdominal surgery. Some techniques that might not exacerbate her condition would be PEP, directed cough (with abdominal support), and flutter.
6. The patient needs to be alert and cooperative. See the procedure in the core text.
7. See Figures 23-4 and 23-5 in the core text.
8. See Figures 23-6 and 23-7 in the core text.
9. IPV and flutter. See the core text for details on how the devices operate.
10. Applies external high-speed vibration to the chest wall. The vibration is transmitted to the airways. See the core text for further details.

REVIEW

True or False

1. True
2. False
3. True
4. False
5. False
6. True
7. True
8. True
9. False
10. True

Multiple Choice

1. d
2. a
3. c

4. b
5. c
6. d

7. d
8. a
9. a

10. a

Lab Activities

1. a. In other words, how do you know when a cough is effective? Can you tell this by simple observation?

   b. If you answered yes to part a of this question, how can you tell?

2. a. Do they use postural drainage and percussion? How about IPV or HFCWO? PEP?

   b. On which patients do they use these techniques?

CHAPTER 24

Discussion Activities and Questions

1. Airway protection and to provide a route for mechanical ventilation.
2. See Figure 24-4 in the core text.
3. Auscultation, chest radiograph, CO_2 detector.
4. The lighted stylet assists in visualization of the airway during intubation.
5. May be inserted without a laryngoscope, may be more stable, easier to provide oral hygiene.
6. See Figures 24-11 and 24-12 in the core text.
7. There are many advantages. Some include less airway resistance, ability to swallow, and ability to speak.
8. Theoretically, the foam cuff will put less pressure on the tracheal wall, thus minimizing tracheal wall damage.
9. Minimal leak technique, minimal occlusion method, and using a cuff manometer. See the core text for additional details.
10. Sufficient length, nonirritating, no sharp edges.

REVIEW

True or False

1. False
2. True
3. True

4. False
5. False
6. True

7. False
8. False
9. True

10. False

Multiple Choice

1. d   3. b   5. c   7. b
2. b   4. a   6. a   8. d

Lab Activities

1. a. More specifically, do they have LMAs, Combitubes, etc.?

   b. Check with the staff and the department procedure manual for guidance.

2. a. Have the tubes been taped? Have they been secured with a commercial device?

   b. You might get some guidance from RTs whom you respect.

3. a. Go to www.youtube.com

   b. Go to www.youtube.com

   c. Go to www.youtube.com

   d. Go to www.youtube.com

4. a. RTs or nursing.

   b. Generally, every shift in most facilities.

   c. RTs or physicians.

   d. Check with the staff.

CHAPTER 25

Discussion Activities and Questions

1. Transpulmonary pressure is often referred to as *alveolar distending pressure*. All of the processes of assisted mechanical ventilation attempt to increase the transpulmonary pressure. During negative pressure ventilation, such as ventilation through a chest cuirass, the ventilator attempts to decrease transpulmonary pressure to enable a larger gas volume to reach the lungs. During positive pressure ventilation, the mechanical ventilator likewise attempts to increase the transpulmonary pressure by delivering a volume of gas to the alveoli.

2. Artificial mechanical ventilation can be administered through three methods: negative pressure ventilation, positive pressure ventilation, and high-frequency ventilation.

3. Airway resistance in the intubated patient can vary for a variety of reasons, such as the diameter of the artificial airway, airway secretions, bronchospasm, pulmonary edema, chronic obstructive pulmonary disease, surfactant deficiency, and any other pathology that creates a high-pressure environment in the lungs. To decrease airway resistance, the clinician needs to correct the problem that is causing the restriction in the lungs.

4. Dynamic compliance (C_{dyn}) measures the changes in volume and pressure in the nonelastic airways. A second type of compliance, known as static compliance (C_{st}), measures the elastic properties of the lungs.

5. One limb utilizes a lower PEEP level and higher F_IO_2. The second limb utilizes a higher PEEP level with a lower F_IO_2.

6. As compliance decreases, the time constant likewise decreases. With a decrease in compliance and time constant, the lung unit loses the potential for reaching its total filling capacity.

7. Decreasing the tidal volume, decreasing the positive end-expiratory pressure, suctioning the patient if the high pressure is a result of secretions, providing bronchodilators if bronchospasm is present, manipulating the inspiratory time.

8. During positive pressure ventilation, the ventilator delivers a volume of gas through either an endotracheal tube or a noninvasive nasal or face mask to the patient's lungs to assist in ventilation. The volume of gas that the ventilator delivers to the lungs causes changes in the alveolar pressure, making the alveolar pressure gradient a positive pressure environment. This positive pressure is transmitted throughout the lungs, and gas exchange results. When an individual is receiving negative pressure ventilation, the upper airway is exposed to ambient pressure while the thoracic cavity is placed in an airtight environment. When negative pressure is applied to this airtight environment, the thoracic cavity pressure drops and becomes a negative pressure environment. In response to the change in thoracic pressure, the intra-alveolar pressure becomes negative as a result of the negative pressure generated at the upper airway.

9. During positive pressure ventilation, the ventilator delivers a volume of gas through either an endotracheal tube or a noninvasive nasal or face mask to the patient's lungs to assist in ventilation. The volume of gas that the ventilator delivers to the lungs causes changes in the alveolar pressure, making the alveolar pressure gradient a positive pressure environment. This positive pressure is transmitted throughout the lungs, and gas exchange results. High-frequency ventilation provides ventilation that delivers a tidal volume less than dead space and respiratory rates anywhere between 60 and 900 breaths per minute.

10. Ventilator-induced injuries, volutrauma, barotrauma, decreased cardiac output.

REVIEW

True or False

1. False
2. True
3. False
4. True
5. True
6. False
7. False
8. False
9. True
10. False

Multiple Choice

1. a
2. c
3. d
4. d
5. a

Lab Activities

1. PIP, PEEP, tidal volume, plateau pressure.

2. Suction, administer bronchodilator.

3. Either limb has been found to be beneficial.

4. Dynamic; it measures the changes in the nonelastic airways.

5. *Volutrauma* is a condition that occurs when too much tidal volume is delivered to the lungs. This large amount of tidal volume has the potential to cause an overdistension of the lungs that results in lung injury. Overdistension can result in stretching of the alveolar spaces, which can lead to an inflammatory mediator release that further injures the lungs. *Barotrauma* results from a high level of positive pressure and causes air to escape from the alveolar areas. Barotrauma results in airleak syndromes such as pneumothorax or pulmonary interstitial emphysema, as well as free air in the thoracic cavity. Both conditions are important because of the potential damage that can occur in the lungs.

CHAPTER 26

Discussion Activities and Questions

1. Apnea, acute ventilatory failure, oxygenation failure, impending ventilatory failure.

2. Any condition that impairs the physiologic pathway of breathing may lead to apnea or acute ventilatory failure, which is the failure of the thorax to pump air.

3. *Oxygenation failure* is the failure of the lungs to provide gas exchange.

4. An extracorporeal membrane oxygenator (ECMO) allows the exchange of O_2 and CO_2 in the blood but does not provide ventilation.

5. The increase in FRC is typically accomplished by applying positive end-expiratory pressure (PEEP). PEEP holds pressure in the lung and increases the end-tidal lung volume.

6. By using PEEP.

7. Physiologic function is often measured to determine the adequacy of a patient's capacity to maintain spontaneous breathing, and to identify impending ventilatory failure. Variables such as vital capacity, negative inspiratory pressure, and maximum voluntary ventilation are typically measured, in addition to arterial blood gases (ABG).

8. Verify ventilator function, select the humidifier type, and connect the humidifier. Calibrate the sensors, set the high airway pressure alarm limit on 40 cm H_2O for *volume control* (*VC*) or on 35 cm H_2O for *volume-targeted pressure control* (*VTPC*). Also for VTPC, set the high tidal volume alarm limit equal to 10 mL/kg. Set a tidal volume (V_T) of 8 mL/kg of *predicted body weight* (*PBW*) at a rate of 15 breaths per minute (bpm). If the plateau pressure is greater than 30 cm H_2O when the ventilator is connected to the patient (low compliance), use 6 mL/kg of PBW V_T and a rate of 20 bpm. If the plateau pressure is still greater than 30 cm H_2O, drop the tidal volume to 4 mL/kg of PBW (minimum tidal volume) and increase the rate to 30 bpm (maximum 35 bpm). Set a peak flow of 50 Lpm or a flow in milliliters per minute equal to V_T mL × bpm × ($I + E$). Set the primary disconnect alarm, the high tidal volume alarm limit, and the apnea ventilation parameters, if available. Set a flow trigger of 2 Lpm. Set 5 cm H_2O PEEP.

9. A ventilator should be on standby, ready for use, and it should have had proper preventative maintenance by qualified staff. Attach a ventilator circuit and connect an appropriate humidification system. Connect the ventilator to a power and gas source. Before the ventilator is connected to the patient, verify its operation and enter the patient values on the control panel. Most ventilators require the selection of the type of humidification system, either a heated wet humidifier or a heat and moisture exchanger (HME), during the initial ventilator startup when the patient's weight is entered. The initial startup is also when flow and oxygen sensors are calibrated and when the neonatal, pediatric, or adult patient range is selected. During this time, the patient is being ventilated with a manual resuscitator or transport ventilator.

    The operation verification procedures vary by ventilator. These programmed self-tests may take several minutes and result in ventilator failure if performed too quickly. Some of the current ventilators have a short leak test, and it should be used. This test creates a pressure hold that checks for leaks, exhalation valve function, and tubing compliance factor. Failure to perform the manufacturer's recommended performance check may cause the ventilator to malfunction during patient use.

10. For older ventilators, the pause pressure generated during the leak test may be used to calculate the circuit compliance or tubing compliance factor.

    - Divide the tidal volume by the pause pressure to calculate the tubing compliance factor.

    - Use this factor to calculate the volume that is compressed in the circuit during a volume-controlled inspiration and that is therefore not delivered to the patient.

    - After the ventilator is connected to the patient, multiply the pressure during a pause (minus any PEEP) by the tubing compliance factor to find the compressible volume loss of the circuit.

- Subtract the compressible volume from the exhaled tidal volume to calculate the tidal volume that the patient actually receives.

Most current critical care ventilators automatically calculate tubing compliance during the performance verification test.

REVIEW

True or False

1. False
2. True
3. True
4. False
5. True
6. True
7. True
8. True
9. True

Multiple Choice

1. d
2. b
3. a
4. d
5. d

CHAPTER 27

Discussion Activities and Questions

1. Three primary variables are assessed with waveforms: pressure, volume, and flow.

2. 7.5

3. 6

4. The positive pressure at the end of exhalation during spontaneous breathing or mechanical ventilation.

5. In a typical volume ventilator breath, the breath begins at a low flow and quickly increases to the set amount, where it is maintained at that constant rate until the end of the inspiratory phase; then exhalation occurs. In a typical pressure-ventilated breath, the breath begins at peak flow and decreases in a linear fashion until the end of inspiration. Exhalation occurs passively at the end of the inspiratory time.

6. Ventilator modes correlate to either pressure or volume. Within the two categories (pressure and volume) are four modes: controlled modes, assist-controlled modes, support modes, and combination modes.
   Controlled modes. In controlled modes, the ventilator starts the breath, controls the inspiratory gas delivery, and ends inspiration with no input from the patient. With each breath is a guaranteed delivery of either a preset pressure or tidal volume that is controlled by the ventilator.
   Assist-controlled modes are identical to control modes except that the patient is able to trigger the ventilator by exerting respiratory muscles.
   Support modes. In support modes, where the patient is breathing spontaneously, the patient initiates the breath and controls the depth of the breath and the flow rate at which the breath is delivered.
   Combination modes include both control (when the patient does not spontaneously initiate a breath) and support (support when the patient breathes spontaneously). It is used primarily to provide partial mechanical support. The patient can take some spontaneous breaths but may also receive some mandatory or control breaths as well.

7. Controlled modes, assist-controlled modes, support modes, and combination modes.

8. Inspiratory is above baseline, expiratory is below baseline.

9. PIP is the highest point, PEEP is the lowest point above the baseline.

10. *Square*—The square scalar waveform is generated by a constant flow rate throughout inspiration. The waveform can also be referred to as a *rectangular* or *constant flow rate wave*.

    Decelerating—The decelerating waveform is generated by flow that begins at peak and decreases in a linear manner until the end of inspiration. This waveform is also known as a *descending waveform*.

    Accelerating—The accelerating waveform is generated by flow that begins with a low level and then increases throughout inspiration. This waveform has also been called an *ascending waveform*.

    Sinusoidal—The sinusoidal waveform is generated by flow that increases to a peak and then decreases. At times only half of this curve may be present.

    Decay—The exponential decay waveform is generated by flow that begins at peak and decreases.

    Rise—The exponential rise waveform is generated by flow that begins at a low level and then increases gradually throughout inspiration.

REVIEW

True or False

1. True
2. True
3. True
4. False
5. False
6. True
7. True
8. True
9. True
10. True

Multiple Choice

1. c
2. b
3. a
4. b
5. d

Lab Activities

1.

Time	Respiratory Rate	TCT
60 sec	60	1
60 sec	30	2
60 sec	20	3
60 sec	15	4
60 sec	12	5
60 sec	10	6
60 sec	6	10

2. First wave is pressure, second wave is flow, third wave is volume.

3. Decelerating waveform.

CHAPTER 28

Discussion Activities and Questions

1. Help improve oxygenation and/or ventilation without having to intubate and mechanically ventilate the patient.

2. Respiratory distress with moderate to severe dyspnea, use of accessory muscles, and abdominal paradox, pH < 7.35 with $PaCO_2$ > 45 mm Hg, A respiratory rate = 25 bpm.

3. In cases of acute respiratory failure, NPPV provides adequate gas exchange and decreased respiratory muscle work without the need for an endotracheal tube or when intubation is undesirable. When applied properly, NPPV of patients with acute exacerbation of COPD reduces mortality and length of intensive care stay. NPPV also reduces the intubation rate in patients with more severe COPD exacerbations. The successful application of NPPV requires the patient to be able to clear secretions effectively.

4. Noninvasive mechanical ventilation includes both positive and negative pressure ventilator applications that do not require the placement of an endotracheal or tracheostomy tube. Invasive ventilation involves using an endotracheal or tracheotomy tube.

5. Altered mental status, ARDS, excessive secretions, extreme anxiety, massive obesity.

6. Burns, facial or skull trauma, hemodynamic instability, need of airway protection, respiratory arrest, uncooperative patient.

7. Noninvasive positive pressure ventilation (NPPV) is a treatment for hypercapnic respiratory failure in which the ventilator-patient interface is typically a nasal mask or an oronasal mask (a mask that covers the nose and mouth). In negative pressure ventilation (NPV), the ventilator is applied to the thorax and abdomen or to the entire body from the neck down, and no ventilator apparatus is in contact with the face. In both types of noninvasive ventilation, gas flows through the upper airway and into the lungs.

8. Inspiratory pressures are increased as needed to achieve a respiratory frequency of less than 25 bpm and a tidal volume of 6–7 mL/kg body weight. Inspiratory pressures of more than 20 cm H_2O may be required, but result in a greater leak. Expiratory pressures are generally 4–8 cm H_2O.

9. IPAP pressures greater than 20 cm H_2O may be required, but may create a greater leak. If higher pressures are needed, check that the mask is the appropriate size. An EPAP pressure of at least 4 cm H_2O reduces the amount of rebreathing. Higher tidal volumes may require a higher level of EPAP to reduce rebreathing. Do not block the exhalation port, and direct it away from the patient's face.

10. Pressure gradient between IPAP and EPAP determines the tidal volume. If EPAP is increased, increase the IPAP by the same amount.

11. NPPV is used primarily for ventilation; CPAP will not improve ventilation, only oxygenation.

REVIEW

True or False

1. False	4. True	7. True	10. False
2. False	5. False	8. False	
3. True	6. True	9. False	

Multiple Choice

1. b
2. d
3. d
4. b
5. d

Lab Activities

1. Main purpose is to treat respiratory failure without the need for invasive ventilation by providing support to decrease PCO_2 levels without using an artificial airway.

2. Several types of NPPV include BiPAP and negative pressure ventilation, which provide ventilation by using positive pressure (BiPAP) and negative pressure.

3. Increasing IPAP will create a bigger pressure gradient, in turn increasing tidal volume for better ventilation. Increasing EPAP will improve oxygenation.

4. IPAP is used for inspiratory pressure; EPAP is used for end expiratory pressure. The gradient between these parameters will help ventilate the patient.

5. BiPAP uses positive pressure ventilation, Pulmo-Wrap uses negative pressure ventilation.

CHAPTER 29

Discussion Activities and Questions

1. *Neonatal* typically refers to the period from birth through the first 4 weeks of life; *pediatric* refers to the period from 1 month to 18 years of age.

2. Clinical studies have shown that delivery room resuscitation with 100% oxygen, when compared with room air, is associated with a lower 5-minute Apgar score, a prolonged time to first cry and breath, increased neonatal mortality, increased oxidative stress (which persisted for at least 4 weeks after birth in one study), increased myocardial and kidney injury, and also a higher risk for childhood leukemia and cancer. These studies were largely undertaken in underdeveloped countries and primarily involved term babies.

   These findings and others have led to the widespread practice of using air-oxygen blenders with resuscitators during delivery. Until the results of further studies become available, a reasonable approach to resuscitation would include initial resuscitation with 30–40% oxygen for very preterm infants, using targeted SpO_2 values and blended oxygen during the first 10 minutes. For ongoing management of preterm infants, SpO_2 targets of 85–93% seem to be most appropriate.

3. In utero, the fetal requirements for oxygen and nutrients are supplied by the oxygenated blood flowing from the placenta to the fetus through the umbilical vein. Carbon dioxide is removed from the fetal blood when it flows back out to the placenta via the umbilical arteries. Fetal cardiac and pulmonary blood flows are different because the fetus needs little blood flow through the lungs. In utero, the resistance to blood flow in the lungs is higher than resistance to blood flow in the rest of the fetus. This causes the majority output of the right ventricle to shunt past the lung directly to the left or somatic side of the cardiac circulation. There are three major sites of shunting: the foramen ovale, the patent ductus arteriosus, and the ductus venosus.

4. Two circumstances are important during the resuscitation of newborns: diaphragmatic hernia and the presence of meconium in the amniotic fluid. In newborns presenting with a diaphragmatic hernia, consider the following:

   • Avoid positive pressure ventilation with a mask; this can force air into the stomach. The stomach and/or small intestines may be extruding into the chest through the defect in the diaphragm. If air is forced into the bowel, the portion of the bowel in the chest cavity can expand and compress other structures in the chest, including the heart, lungs, and great vessels. If positive pressure ventilation is needed (which is likely in diaphragmatic hernia), the patient should be intubated as soon after delivery as possible to avoid distension of the bowel.

- A newborn might have meconium in the amniotic fluid at delivery: *Meconium* is a thick, dark, viscous fluid that is a waste product of the fetal bowel and that normally occurs in trace amounts in the amniotic fluid. It is nearly sterile but can be chemically irritating to the lung. When the infant is stressed during labor and delivery, the bowel can evacuate in utero and the amniotic fluid can contain varying amounts of meconium, which can then be aspirated into the infant's upper airway. If it is, it can cause obstruction of the airways and chemical irritation of the airways and lung tissue (*meconium aspiration syndrome*). This syndrome, in its severe forms, can be life threatening. During labor, the amniotic fluid is examined and tested for meconium staining. If thick meconium is present, the clinician who delivers the infant should suction the upper airway when the head is delivered, prior to delivery of the rest of the infant's body. After delivery of the rest of the body, the infant is intubated and immediately suctioned—if possible, before initiating the first breath by the infant. If the meconium staining is mild, it is usually necessary only to thoroughly suction the upper airway.

5. Clinical scoring systems now abound in the hospital. There are asthma scores, bronchiolitis scores, coma scores, and trauma scores. All these scores help in bringing a degree of sorely needed standardization to the way clinicians evaluate patients. A pioneer in this field in the early 1950s, Dr. Virginia Apgar created a simple yet reliable and effective method of assessing the cardiorespiratory status of infants at delivery and of assessing the effectiveness of resuscitation efforts. The scoring is done by evaluating the patient for five signs: heart rate, color, respiratory effort, muscle tone, and reflex irritability.

6. Apgar scores are typically assessed at 1 and 5 minutes after delivery by the respiratory therapist, nurse, or doctor participating in the resuscitation. The scoring is done by evaluating the patient for five signs: heart rate, color, respiratory effort, muscle tone, and reflex irritability; these are related to how the infant reacts to stimuli. An ordinal score of 0, 1, or 2 is assigned to each of these categories and then totaled.

7. *Pneumothorax* is leakage and dissection of air into the pleural space. If air continues to accumulate, causing significant compression of adjacent lung tissues and vascular structure, it is called a *tension pneumothorax*. Small pneumothoraces may resolve spontaneously, but larger pneumothoraces require evacuation of the air in the pleural cavity via chest tube. A tension pneumothorax happens almost exclusively during positive pressure ventilation. During inspiration, the positive pressure forces air out through the site(s) of the leak. It is assumed that during exhalation, these leak sites close so that this pressurized air accumulates in the pleural space with each successive breath. Untreated, the tension pneumothorax may be immediately life threatening because it can grow so large that it compresses lung tissue and vascular structures in the thorax.

8. There are three major sites of shunting: the foramen ovale, the patent ductus arteriosus, and the ductus venosus.

- The *foramen ovale* is a flaplike opening between the right and left atria, allowing blood flow only from the right to the left side of the heart under normal conditions.

- The *ductus arteriosus* is a connection between the ascending aorta and the pulmonary artery.

- The *ductus venosus* connects the umbilical vein directly to the inferior vena cava, allowing most blood to bypass the liver.

9. Maternal factors that can lead to premature birth include:

- High blood pressure of pregnancy, also known as *pre-eclampsia* or *toxemia* of pregnancy.

- Infections of the fetal/placental tissues, vagina, or urinary tract.

- Drug use.

- Abnormal uterine morphology.

- Inability of the cervix to stay closed during pregnancy (also known as *cervical incompetence*).

10. The causes of ROP are multifactorial, and oxygenation derangement alone does not explain the pathology. But oxygen therapy plays a major role, and the RT treating the low-birth-weight/premature infant has an important role in keeping blood oxygen levels within a "safe" range to reduce the risk of ROP. Generally accepted treatment guidelines include keeping PaO_2 in the range of 50–90 mm Hg or SpO_2 in the range of 88–94%.

REVIEW

True or False

1. True	4. True	7. True	10. True
2. True	5. True	8. True	
3. True	6. True	9. True	

Multiple Choice

1. d	3. d	5. b
2. d	4. d	

Lab Activities

1. Misconception: *Neonatal and pediatric practice is harder or more demanding than respiratory care for adult populations.*

   Truth: These respective practice environments are simply different. So, to practice effectively in most neonatal and pediatric populations, the respiratory therapist needs different preparation, training, and experience than respiratory therapists who treat adult populations.

   Misconception: *Pediatric patients are small adults, and neonates are smaller pediatric patients.*

   Truth: Nothing could be further from the truth. For example, a premature neonate is indeed very small, but also has tissues and organ systems in various stages of development. Depending on the patient's gestational age at birth, some organ systems can be very underdeveloped, particularly the lungs in babies born under 35 weeks of gestation. In general, the airways form early in gestational life (by about 17 weeks) and grow by enlargement. At the same time, the alveoli develop late in gestational life and early childhood and grow by forming new structures. At term, the healthy newborn has approximately 150 million alveoli, although this number is highly variable. Apparently, new alveolar structures are added throughout the first few years of life (for a total of about 274–790 million), and further lung growth takes place by enlargement of the existing structure.

2. Normally, blood flow through the fetal heart and lungs is different when in the uterus than in the neonate after delivery. During the delivery and in the immediate postnatal period, the newborn must transition from having gas exchange supported mostly by the mother's cardiac output to completely independent breathing and adult patterns of blood flow. Failure to make a rapid transition can result in life-threatening conditions, such as persistent pulmonary hypertension of the newborn.

   In utero, the fetal requirements for oxygen and nutrients are supplied by the oxygenated blood flowing from the placenta to the fetus through the umbilical vein. Carbon dioxide is removed from the fetal blood when it flows back out to the placenta via the umbilical arteries. Fetal cardiac and pulmonary blood flows are different because the fetus needs little blood flow through the lungs. In utero, the resistance to blood flow in the lungs is higher than resistance to blood flow in the rest of the fetus. This causes the majority output of the right ventricle to shunt past the lung directly to the left or somatic side of the cardiac circulation. There are three major sites of shunting: the foramen ovale, the patent ductus arteriosus, and the ductus venosus.

Normal fetal PaO₂ is 25–35 mm Hg. This is possible because the fetus is in a nearly motionless state and in a neutral thermal environment; it needs less oxygen to maintain body temperature and muscle activity. Also, a fetus has predominantly *fetal* hemoglobin. This variant of adult hemoglobin has a higher affinity for oxygen at lower PaO₂. This fetal hemoglobin is normally replaced by adult hemoglobin shortly after birth. After the clamping of the umbilical vessels, the low-resistance circulatory system of the placenta is removed from the fetal circulation.

- As the lungs inflate and gas exchange occurs, an increase in PaO₂ causes dilation of the pulmonary arterial bed, resulting in a reduction in pulmonary vascular resistance (PVR).

- Blood pressure in the right (or pulmonary) side of the heart decreases relative to the blood pressure in the left or somatic side of the heart.

- The pressure in the aorta increases and becomes greater than the pressure in the pulmonary artery. This decreases the amount of right-to-left shunting through the ductus arteriosus and foramen ovale.

- Closure of the ductus arteriosus usually occurs within the first 24 hours to 2 weeks of life, except in the premature infant, in whom musculature of the ductus arteriosus may not be well developed and thus its ability to constrict may be limited. The PVR is lower than the systemic vascular resistance (SVR), and blood flows into the lungs from the systemic circulation (left to right). The ductus arteriosus may not close completely in some term infants (e.g., in meconium aspiration). These patients may experience very high PVR, and blood then flows from right to left through the ductus arteriosus from the pulmonary circulation to the systemic circulation, bypassing the lungs. Because the foramen ovale flap allows blood to flow only from right to left, it closes when the pressures in the LA become greater than those in the RA. If the foramen ovale lacks a flap-like structure or has a defective one, the opening begins to function as an *atrial septal defect* (*ASD*).

3. Neutral thermal environment, insensible water loss, and minimal stimulation.

    Low-birth-weight infants are fragile and delicate. They do not tolerate excessive handling well. They are very sensitive to changes in ambient temperature. They have very little physiologic reserve; when stressed, they can have a profound response, which usually manifests itself in hypoxemia and/or bradycardia. Newborns and particularly premature infants are at risk of severe physiologic insult if careful attention is not paid to maintaining their body temperature. Premature newborns are soon placed under radiant warmers or in incubators, which limit heat loss by providing a neutral thermal environment around the patient.

4. Two circumstances are important during the resuscitation of newborns: diaphragmatic hernia and the presence of meconium in the amniotic fluid. A newborn might have meconium in the amniotic fluid at delivery: *Meconium* is a thick, dark, viscous fluid that is a waste product of the fetal bowel and that normally occurs in trace amounts in the amniotic fluid. It is nearly sterile but can be chemically irritating to the lung. When the infant is stressed during labor and delivery, the bowel can evacuate in utero and the amniotic fluid can contain varying amounts of meconium, which can then be aspirated into the infant's upper airway. If it is, it can cause obstruction of the airways and chemical irritation of the airways and lung tissue (*meconium aspiration syndrome*). This syndrome, in its severe forms, can be life threatening. During labor, the amniotic fluid is examined and tested for meconium staining. If thick meconium is present, the clinician who delivers the infant should suction the upper airway when the head is delivered, prior to delivery of the rest of the infant's body. After delivery of the rest of the body, the infant is intubated and immediately suctioned—if possible, before initiating the first breath by the infant. If the meconium staining is mild, it is usually necessary only to thoroughly suction the upper airway.

5. The two principal parts of this respiratory assessment are a visual inspection and auscultation. In addition to the previously described signs associated with assessing respiratory failure in infants, a special consideration for the respiratory assessment of infants and children is the use (or lack of use) of blood gases. The other key factors in respiratory assessment are:

- Respiratory rate
- Grunting
- Flaring
- Retracting
- Level of consciousness
- Level of irritation

CHAPTER 30

Discussion Activities and Questions

1. Older people and minorities tend to use more health-care resources.

2. *Part A.* Hospital insurance; also covers skilled nursing facilities, hospice, and home health care under certain conditions.

   Part B. Medical insurance; helps cover medically necessary services such as physician's services and out-patient care. Some preventative services are also covered.

3. They may have more health problems than younger patients. They may have sensory deficits that make it more difficult for them to follow instructions. They may have mental issues (e.g., dementia) that make it more difficult for them to be cooperative.

4. The elderly are frequently victims of many chronic illnesses. Some of these include COPD, CHF, Parkinson's, and Alzheimer's. See Table 30-3 in the core text.

5. See Tables 30-4 and 30-5 in the core text.

6. Turning up the volume on the television, straining to hear conversation (among others).

7. Decrease extraneous noise; face patient when speaking; use more visual aids.

8. See Table 30-6 in the core text.

9. Medications, lack of exercise, disease processes.

10. Lack of financial resources, use of nonprescription drugs, nutritional deficits, decreased cognitive ability.

Thought Questions

1. Do you have aging parents or grandparents? What health issues are they facing? If you do not personally know anyone who is over the age of 65, think about the patients you have seen in the hospital.

2. Hospital patients tend to look older than they really are; likewise for people with chronic diseases.

3. Go back and review the tables of ADLs and IADLs. Contact a local senior center for guidance, if you do not know any elderly persons.

4. This is a difficult situation. Does the patient live alone, or does he have people around him? He needs to be educated about both the inhaler and the concentrator.

5. Presence of potential caregivers, adequate electrical supply, decreased clutter, presence of pets (cats in particular may chew on the tubing), access to communication device (e.g., telephone), hygiene, distance between important areas of the home (e.g., bathroom, bed, kitchen, etc.). To correct any deficiencies, you might have to contact social services in your area.

6. The AARC has published a guide to aerosol use that includes the cost of inhalers. Go the AARC website (www.aarc.org) for further details. You could also use webMD or some other popular website to find information about drug prices.

7. If possible, check the medical record. Do not breach any confidentiality in the process.

REVIEW

True or False

1. True
2. False
3. False
4. False
5. True
6. True
7. False
8. True
9. False
10. True

Multiple Choice

1. b
2. c
3. b
4. b
5. a

CHAPTER 31

Discussion Activities and Questions

1. Assuming that the patient is breathing, place the patient on his or her side (see the core text for more details).

2. Primarily, inability to speak, clutching throat, appearing to panic.

3. Family history of heart disease, risky behaviors (e.g., cigarette smoking), lack of exercise, high stress (among others).

4. Basic life support is supportive care: compressions, ventilation, and defibrillation (if indicated). In ACLS, an attempt is made to find the cause of the arrest and correct it. ACLS also includes other cardiac anomalies (e.g., symptomatic bradycardia, etc.). In addition, consider the placement of advanced airways.

5. There are current differences between the two. Also, the biphasic defibrillator tends to use less energy (as measured in joules).

6. During a chaotic rescue attempt, it is very difficult for the rescuers (especially the charge person) to remember what has happened. The scribe is essential in recording each action as it occurs. The scribe may also keep track of the time. Finally, the scribe provides documentation of the rescue attempt.

7. Cardioversion may be done in cases of ventricular tachycardia where the patient has a pulse. It also provides a shock; however, it synchronizes the shock with the patient's QRS.

8. The advantages of automated defibrillators are obvious. However, during an extended ACLS-type code, it is crucial to put the decision to defibrillate into the hands of an experienced team leader.

9. Apnea, asystole, bradycardia, extreme cyanosis, flaccid and unresponsive to stimuli, secondary apnea.

10. The basic equipment is pretty much the same (ET tube, laryngoscope, etc.). See the core text for more details.

REVIEW

True or False

1. True
2. False
3. True
4. True
5. False
6. False
7. False
8. True
9. True
10. False

Multiple Choice

1. a	4. a	7. c	10. b
2. d	5. d	8. c	
3. a	6. c	9. c	

Lab Activities

1. The 2010 guidelines can be accessed at http://circ.ahajournals.org/content/122/18_suppl_3.toc. The 2005 guidelines can be accessed at http://circ.ahajournals.org/content/112/24_suppl.toc

2. This is a difficult question to answer. However, one thing you must accept is that the person in charge is the one who makes the ultimate decision. If you do not agree with the decision, you can voice your opinion. But in the end, you should support the decision that is made.

4. See the 2010 guidelines. The algorithms are basically the same, with some slight modifications of the compression and ventilation rates.

CHAPTER 32

Discussion Activities and Questions

1. Hospitals should have an incident command system. See the core text for further details.

2. Disasters such as earthquakes, hurricanes, and tornadoes. One might also consider human-caused disasters, such as massive explosions.

3. There would be many types of injuries following an earthquake. Some of these would include crush injuries. However, you might also expect to see inhalation and burn injuries, among many others.

4. The blast lung triad is the result of a blast injury. Look for respiratory distress, bat-wing appearance on chest film, and hypoxia.

5. Primarily respiratory precautions.

6. Clear sensorium, afebrile, symmetrical descending paralysis.

7. Support the medical team, protect the airway, and provide ventilatory support as necessary.

8. Mass casualties with minimal or no trauma; first responders are also casualties; dead animals and/or vegetation in the area.

9. The antidote is sodium nitrite.

10. Epidemics result from infectious diseases that spread through a local population. *Pandemics* are enlarged epidemics.

Thought Questions

1. a. Obviously, the answer will depend on the movies chosen. However, most movie disasters are things like earthquakes, tornadoes, or explosions. These will result first in bodily injuries progressing to lung injuries.

   b. Every hospital should have a disaster plan in place in order to deal with anticipated mass casualties.

3. Although answers will be specific to individual student and area, to be well prepared for a bioterrorist attack, a hospital should have a well-developed disaster plan in place.

4. In recent years, hospitals have had to develop plans to deal with outbreaks of various influenza strains. One of the parts of the planning process has been to increase the number of ventilators on hand.

REVIEW

True or False

1. False
2. True
3. True
4. False
5. True
6. False
7. False
8. True
9. False
10. True

Multiple Choice

1. b
2. c
3. a
4. d
5. d

CHAPTER 33

Discussion Activities and Questions

1. Acute Physiology and Chronic Health Evaluation (APACHE) II includes 12 physiological variables. Sequential organ failure assessment (SOFA) utilizes the assessment of six organ systems. See the core text for additional details.

2. *Care plans* are written instructions and guidelines for the care of patients who have specific disorders. These plans are used primarily to provide consistent and uniform care.

3. To monitor the nutritional status of patients in critical care.

4. Making the transition from complete ventilatory support to spontaneous breathing requires adequate nutrition as fuel. A patient who is poorly nourished (i.e., has insufficient caloric support) is less likely to wean successfully.

5. Closed, open, and co-managed. See the core text for details.

6. Think of the skills you are learning as a respiratory therapist. Some of these applied to critical care are mechanical ventilation, inhaled medication delivery, and oxygen therapy.

7. As an RT, you are a health-care professional, and thus bear an extra burden of responsibility. Some skills for which you might be cross-trained are venipuncture, 12-lead ECG, IV management, arterial line management, and acute cardiac care (e.g., intra-aortic balloon pump management).

8. As medicine becomes more evidence based, you should become familiar with levels of evidence (generally obtained during clinical studies). Level I is the highest level, usually obtained during double-blind, placebo controlled, multicenter trials.

9. A *protocol* is an algorithm that leads to appropriate therapy for a patient. A *clinical practice guideline* is an evidence-driven statement on how a particular therapeutic modality should be used.

10. Suctioning and arterial blood gas analysis.

Thought Questions

1. Check with the RT department medical director.

2. Check with nursing for the care plans; they may also be computer generated.

3. What do these flow sheets have in common? How often are ventilator checks done in each hospital?

REVIEW

True or False

1. True

2. False

3. True

4. True

5. False

6. False

7. True

8. True

Multiple Choice

1. b

2. d

3. c

4. d

5. d

CHAPTER 34

Discussion Activities and Questions

1. Goal-oriented treatment.

2. Many chronic conditions that have created disability or debility in a patient (e.g., COPD, quadriplegia, etc.). Some patients might also be recovering from surgery or bone fractures (e.g., rehab following hip surgery).

3. Subacute facilities will have probably have expanded physical and occupational therapy. They may also have other therapies, such as recreational. They can be very rehabilitation oriented.

4. *Nursing homes* are residences for people who can no longer care for themselves. *Skilled nursing facilities* are facilities that handle long-term, complex medical conditions and provide rehab services.

5. *Case management* is a method of medical management in which a person—the case manager—is assigned patients who have the same types of problems, to standardize care.

6. The Muse report indicated that respiratory therapists provide high-quality care with definite positive patient outcomes.

7. See Table 34-1 in the core text.

8. One way is that there are generally fewer personnel (especially physicians) on duty 24 hours a day. A second way is that there is less monitoring and less complex resource utilization.

9. At minimum, the patient will need tracheostomy care, suction equipment, some kind of humidification for the trach when he is not on the ventilator, and a ventilator that does not take up too much space. The caregivers will need instruction and certification of competency.

10. The main differences relate to reimbursement, licensing, services offered, and types of residents.

Thought Question

4. The initial assessment should include a thorough respiratory exam, including SpO_2 and auscultation, plus a history. This should be done upon admission.

REVIEW

True or False

1. True
2. False
3. False
4. True
5. True

Multiple Choice

1. a
2. c
3. a
4. b
5. d

CHAPTER 35

Discussion Activities and Questions

1. The goal of home respiratory care is to achieve the optimum level of patient function through goal setting, education, the administration of diagnostic and therapeutic modalities and services, disease management, and health promotion.

2. See Table 35-1 in the core text.

3. A patient qualifies for home oxygen (according to Medicare guidelines) if the PaO_2 is 55 mm Hg or less, or the SpO_2 is 88% or less. The testing must be done with the patient on room air at rest.

4. See Figure 35-1 and refer to the explanation in the core text.

5. See Figure 35-3 and refer to the core text for additional explanation.

6. See Table 35-6 and refer to the core text for additional details.

7. The types of bronchial hygiene most likely to be used in the home are high-frequency chest wall oscillation ("The Vest"), flutter, and postural drainage and percussion.

8. • Obstructive sleep apnea with CPAP treatment has been ruled out.

   • Either an arterial PCO_2 from a blood gas test is equal to or greater than 52 mm Hg (done while the patient was awake and breathing the usual F_IO_2), or an oxygen saturation is equal to or less than 88% during sleep for at least 5 continuous minutes while the patient is breathing the usual F_IO_2 or 2 Lpm, whichever is higher. Also see Table 35-10 in the core text.

9. The three alarms are bradycardia, tachycardia, and apnea.

10. The Joint Commission sets standards by which HMEs are evaluated. This provides assurance and uniformity for the public.

Thought Questions

1. Reimbursement is a serious issue in home care. The best way you can help the reimbursement situation is to support AARC initiatives to increase Medicare recognition of respiratory care.

2. Besides the usual competencies in basic respiratory care, the home care RT should also possess excellent assessment and communication skills.

3. One way would be to communicate frequently with the patient and the patient's family. Some CPAP units have the ability to monitor compliance with built-in chips. You could also monitor health care resource utilization.

4. There are advantages of and disadvantages to each type of humidification. However, for portable ventilation, HMEs are probably more practical.

5. Mostly, SpO_2. You could also monitor breath sounds.

6. You would certainly monitor and assess the home environment for various forms of safety (e.g., electrical). You would also want to monitor hygiene and caregiver support.

REVIEW

True or False

1. True	4. True	7. False	10. False
2. False	5. True	8. False	11. True
3. False	6. False	9. True	

Multiple Choice

1. a	3. a	5. c
2. c	4. d	

CHAPTER 36

Discussion Activities and Questions

1. *Pulmonary rehabilitation* is a program of education and exercise that focuses on restoring chronic respiratory patients to the highest functional capacity possible.

    Cardiac rehabilitation is a comprehensive education and exercise program designed to improve the cardiovascular fitness of patients with known cardiac dysfunction.

2. See Figure 36-1 in the core text.

3. *Abnormal pulmonary mechanics* often results in increased respiratory muscle work for a set level of ventilation.

4. The point at which the carbon dioxide production equals oxygen consumption.

5. Respiratory rate, tidal volume, minute volume, anaerobic threshold, dead space to tidal volume ratio, respiratory quotient (among others).

6. PFT, ABGs, ECG, patient history (among others).

7. The closed format uses a set period of time with a designated number of class sessions and a specific end date. *Open-format programs*, in contrast, have no designated number of class sessions or specific end dates. See also Table 36-3 in the core text.

8. Oxygen delivery devices, nebulizers, incentive spirometers (for breathing retraining), batteries (for portable monitoring devices), tissues, cups (among others). These are commonly used and will be needed for patient education and training.

9. Diaphragmatic breathing helps with breath control and panic control; it also helps to use principal muscles of ventilation. Pursed-lip breathing provides a small amount of back pressure to keep the airways open during exhalation.

10. Proper nutrition to maintain adequate body weight (especially important in COPD). Panic control (patients with chronic respiratory diseases tend to panic when short of breath). Lifestyle management to assist in coping with disability. Appropriate medication use.

Thought Questions

1. Access the Borg scale at www.chronicconditions.org/clearinghouse/doc/borg_scale.doc. It probably could be applied to hospitalized patients.

2. a. You will need all the resources listed in the core text, especially equipment and physical space.

   b. Reimbursement should be available through Medicare Part B or private insurance. You would need to investigate the mechanics of how these reimbursement plans operate.

3. Besides being a skilled and competent respiratory therapist, the rehab specialist needs excellent assessment and communication skills. He or she also needs teaching and management skills.

4. As you assess and interact with patients who are suffering from chronic lung diseases, you could at least mention the pulmonary rehab program and indicate how you think they would benefit from it.

REVIEW

True or False

1. False
2. False
3. True
4. True
5. True
6. False
7. True
8. False
9. True
10. False

Multiple Choice

1. a
2. d
3. d
4. a
5. d

CHAPTER 37

Discussion Activities and Questions

1. Advance planning, pretransport assessment, communication, equipment, identification of hazards.

2. Clinical status, excessive vibration (among others).

3. Intrahospital transport is a relatively common occurrence. A critically ill patient might be transferred from a unit to surgery or from the ED to the ICU. Such a patient might also be transported to other departments for testing (e.g., MRI, CT, etc.).

4. You should probably postpone transport until the patient is more stable. Ventricular tachycardia is a life-threatening arrhythmia.

5. You would recognize this by observing the ventilator/patient interaction (i.e., monitor the ventilator function and also monitor patient response and chest rise). The first step when experiencing a ventilator malfunction is to remove the patient from the ventilator and provide manual ventilation.

Thought Questions

2. Factors include portable oxygen (e.g., E cylinder), portable ventilator or hand resuscitator, and a ventilator that is compatible with MRI.

REVIEW

True or False

1. False
2. True
3. False
4. True
5. False
6. False
7. True

Multiple Choice

1. d
2. b
3. d
4. a
5. c

CHAPTER 38

Discussion Activities and Questions

1. The spread of infectious disease requires six elements, called the *chain of infection:* infectious agent, reservoir, portal of exit, method of transmission, portal of entry, susceptible host. See the core text for further details.

2. It is much more likely to cause disease.

3. A *case* is a person who is symptomatic with an illness; for example, a person with pneumonia. A *carrier* is a person who is infected with and can transmit a disease but has no signs or symptoms of the disease.

4. A *vector* is any organism that carries a pathogen from one host to another.

5. See Table 38-2 in the core text.

6. Hand hygiene is one of the most important things a caregiver can do to minimize the spread of infection. See the core text for more details.

7. See Figure 38-4 in the core text.

8. See Table 38-9 in the core text.

9. VRE and MRSA.

10. See Table 38-10 in the core text.

Thought Questions

1. Check with each individual clinic site; however, most large equipment must be surface disinfected only.

2. a. Think contact or airborne isolation. Also, do not forget reverse isolation.

   b. Read the instructions that should be posted on the patient's room door. What kind of isolation is the patient in?

4. a. Although answers will be specific to individual student and area, hospital policies usually are very clear on how to avoid sharps injuries. Be sure to be familiar with these policies.

   b. Although answers will be specific to individual student and area, hospitals usually accommodate latex-intolerant health-care workers by providing latex-free equipment (especially gloves).

   c. Familiarize yourself with the VAP bundle that appears earlier in the core text. Also, always practice good hand hygiene.

REVIEW

True or False

1. True	4. False	7. False	10. False
2. True	5. True	8. True	11. True
3. False	6. False	9. False	

Multiple Choice

1. d	3. b	5. c
2. d	4. c	

CHAPTER 39

Discussion Activities and Questions

1. The World Health Organization came out with a revised and more comprehensive definition of *health*, defining it as "a state of complete physical, mental, and social well-being and not merely the absence of disease or infirmity."

2. There are multiple factors, starting with genetics; others include diet, lifestyle, and one's view of life. See the core text for more details.

3. *Morbidity* is defined as the ratio of persons who are diseased to those who are well in a given community. *Mortality* is defined as the number of deaths per unit of population in a specific region, age range, or other group. Both mortality and morbidity have gone down over the past century.

4. *Wellness* has been expressed as "an approach to personal health that emphasizes individual responsibility for well-being through the practice of health-promoting lifestyle behaviors."

5. Intellectually well people use the intellectual and cultural activities in and beyond the classroom, combined with the human and learning resources available within their community.

6. At least in American culture, there is a tendency to overeat at social functions and a tendency to stress being very productive (thus leading to sleep deprivation and stress). See the core text for more details.

7. Coronary artery disease, various forms of cancer (especially lung cancer), COPD, and diabetes (among others).

8. • Inadequacies in the existing health-care system

   • Behavioral factors or unhealthy lifestyles

   • Environmental hazards

   • Human biological factors

9. See Figure 39-5 in the core text.

10. See Table 39-7 in the core text and text related to *Healthy People 2010*.

Thought Questions

1. a. Although answers will be specific to individual student and area, patients with medical conditions often appear older than their chronological age.

   b. Patients with medical conditions often share the traits of either poor genetics (e.g., people with heart disease frequently have immediate family member who suffer from heart disease) or poor lifestyle choices (e.g.. cigarette smoking).

2. a. Can you get more exercise, get more quality sleep, reduce factors that contribute to poor health?

   b. Model healthy behavior.

3. See Table 39-3 in the core text for the models. At present, medicine seems oriented primarily toward the medical model. Does this seem right to you?

6. The medical model relies heavily on medication. However, there are other things you can try, such as counseling.

REVIEW

True or False

1. False
2. True
3. False

4. True
5. True
6. False

7. True
8. False
9. False

10. True

Multiple Choice

1. a
2. c

3. c
4. d

5. d

CHAPTER 40

Discussion Activities and Questions

1. The learner learns *what* the learner wants to learn *when* the learner *wants* to learn it. This is one of the basic precepts of adult education and probably does apply to students.

2. A *goal* is a general statement of purpose, and it is usually a simple item that may be measured to determine the success of a plan.

3. Informally, the educator can simply ask questions that address the expectations for the patient after the learning process is completed.

4. Communication in patient education is predominately interpersonal in nature. It involves a series of behaviors that are specifically verbal and nonverbal and that stimulate personal inquiry between two or more persons.

5. Reflecting and inventory questioning permit educators to direct feedback to learners regarding how the educators' messages are being received. See the core text for examples.

6. Adult orientation to learning is life centered; therefore, the appropriate units for organizing adult learning are life situations, not subjects.

7. • *Precontemplative.* The patient may not be aware of or even considering a change.

   • *Contemplative.* The patient begins thinking about changes but is not yet taking any action.

   • *Action.* The patient has begun to make changes to behavior and is now practicing the different behaviors.

   • *Maintenance.* The patient has retained the behavior either by learning or via reinforcement.

   • *Termination.* Intervention for the patient has ended, and the behavior has become a way of life and is no longer visualized or perceived by the patient as a change.

8. You can question the patient, ask for a return demonstration, or ask the patient's caregivers.

9. "Training the Health-Care Professional for the Role of Patient and Caregiver Educator."

10. Actually, there are many that are specific to respiratory care. Two include disease education (specifically on asthma and COPD) and smoking cessation.

11. They may not be specific to the topic. The reading level might not be appropriate for the patient population.

Thought Questions

1. [Answers will be specific to individual student.]

2. A placebo (or the patient's real) inhaler would be very useful, along with a valved holding chamber. A quiet location would also be useful. You should plan on taking at least 10 to 15 minutes (long enough for instruction and a return instruction). Your approach would depend largely on the clinical context. Ideally, the patient's parents or guardians should also be present.

3. The patient will probably be placed on CPAP for the sleep apnea. Think in terms of both being familiar and comfortable with the equipment and also understanding the need for the treatment.

4. Remember that the objectives should contain action verbs and be measurable (e.g., "The patient will be able to successfully execute all the steps required to actuate the metered dose inhaler").

5. You might be able to find such examples at the nurses' station or in the respiratory department. Evaluate for such things as readability and use of color and graphics.

6. Some topics might include oxygen delivery devices, respiratory diseases, or inhaled medication. To proceed, go through the steps involved in setting up an appropriate education session.

REVIEW

True or False

1. True	4. True	7. False	10. True
2. False	5. True	8. False	
3. False	6. False	9. True	

Multiple Choice

1. b	3. d	5. c
2. a	4. b	

CHAPTER 41

Discussion Activities and Questions

1. The *medical director* is the individual who has direct responsibility for the quality of patient care.

2. *Centralized* means that the respiratory care department is an autonomous department within the hospital or nursing home. *Decentralized* denotes a structure in which respiratory care personnel report directly to a patient care area such as a nursing unit.

3. A *service line* is a product or service that the department offers. These might include ventilatory support, patient education, and aerosol therapy.

4. These might be items such as oxygen delivery devices, nebulizers, and ventilator circuits.

5. A purchasing group has the advantage of large-volume, bulk purchasing and thus may be able to negotiate better pricing.

6. Decreased hospital days and gatekeeping. See the core text for details.

7. Working conditions, advancement potential, benefits.

8. The discipline of employees is highly important to the successful manager and leader because the process reinforces the need for employees to follow standards.

9. Faster, more reliable communication and documentation, less paper, increased accountability (see the core text for more details).

Thought Questions

1. Check with the department manager or supervisor. You could also check the department policy and procedure manual.

2. How are therapist assignments routinely made? Where are the therapists routinely stationed?

3. Are some (or all) of the therapists skilled in cardiovascular areas (e.g., 12-lead ECG monitoring)?

4. Are they written out at the beginning of the shift? Who makes the assignments? Are the assignments computer generated?

5. Check the department policy and procedure manual. How does the department prepare for Joint Commission surveys?

6. Do they have a computer system for tracking productivity, or is it written out? Do the RTs need to keep track of and report all of the procedures they perform during their shifts?

7. This is a difficult question that the profession has been grappling with for many years. Look at the RTs you have been in contact with. What degrees do they hold? Where did they get their degrees?

8. You have to answer this question for yourself. Assuming that you have had at least one job in your life, what factors have motivated you?

REVIEW

True or False

1. True	4. False	7. False	10. True
2. True	5. False	8. False	
3. False	6. True	9. False	

Multiple Choice

1. a	3. b	5. a
2. d	4. c	